Acknowledgements...

At times our own light goes out and is rekindled by a spark from another person. Each of us has cause to think with deep gratitude of those who have lighted the flame within us. ~Albert Schweitzer

I had no idea until I started this book how many people I was indebted to. I could go on thanking people right here until you put the book down and walk away,. So to avoid overdoing the thanks, I will just stick to the people who helped make this book a reality.

First and foremost, I have to thank Meyrick Jones. You will learn more about him in the book ahead, like the fact that I never would have made the transition to being fit without him. I hope everyone is lucky enough to have friends as supportive as Meyrick.

I am also indebted to the great trainers I had at Innovative Fitness. You did so much more than just teach me how to exercise properly-with an intensity necessary to excel-you also helped me to understand how to take control of my life along with my fitness. I would like to say a huge thank you to Innovative Fitness itself, an unbelievably great business, that has at it's core, the goal of helping people change their lives. I can't think of many businesses that have such a grand purpose, and none that achieve their purpose with such excellence.

I owe a huge thank you to my brother Jeff Vaughan for all of those days talking about health and fitness, comparing notes on our weight loss, and competing in diets and exercise plans. Much of the information in this book came directly from those sessions.

Thank you to Robert Battiston for getting me out on all of those bike rides and for forcing me to try to join Masters Swim Class, something I never would have done without you dragging me over to meet the teacher. Thank you Jason Clement, for helping me continue to set goals and achieve them. As well, thanks for being my Injury Prevention Coach. At first I just thought this was a funny title, but over the last few years, I have come to appreciate how hard it is to keep from injuring yourself because you always think you are fitter than you are.

When the book was complete...the first time, I sent a copy to Wayne Elwood, who makes an appearance in Chapter 5. It turns out Wayne is an editor and he helped turn my rambling thoughts into a more cohesive guide on learning about fit people. Thank you so much Wayne, it was a lot of work to turn it around, but I think it was worth it.

Thank you to everyone who gave the book a read through, especially in the early days. This list includes Michelle, Carolyn, Patty, and Jason. All of your advice helped to make this book better and all of your encouragement helped to make it a reality.

Finally, a thank you to my family. Taylor and Kayley, this book was actually written while you guys learned to sleep through the night and I sat out in the hallway with my laptop. I really never would have gotten my thoughts down without this time to focus. Michelle, thank you for putting up with the hours that I have spent sitting on the computer working on this project. It was so much more than just writing a book, it required a ton of work, as I learned. Thanks mom and dad for always being so supportive of me. It really is amazing what you can achieve when you have the support of your friends and family.

Megan Cole.

Chapter 1
The day my world changed...

He who would learn to fly one day must first learn to stand and walk and run and climb and dance; one cannot fly into flying. ~Friedrich Nietzsche

I will never forget that day. Standing in my bathroom after getting out of the shower about 30 pounds and 6 years ago. I might have considered getting on the scale, but I knew I was well overweight, and I had a pretty good idea of what the scale would say. The past 8 or so years had not been kind to me, as I had gained weight every year.

I had been trying to lose weight since my early twenties, when I started ballooning up for no good reason. I hadn't changed what I was eating or drinking, at least not that I was aware of. But still, while all of my friends watched with amusement, I got fatter and fatter.

So, over the years I dieted and got fatter, and on this morning I stood in the bathroom realizing that I was part of this epidemic of weight gain in North America. I had tried to be fit. I had joined a gym, I had bought expensive exercise equipment, I had reduced my fat intake and nothing was working. The weirdest part of this was that up until this moment, I didn't think I was like every other overweight person out there. I was different. They weren't trying, I was. They were dumb and lazy, and I wasn't. It was then that I realized that if all of the things that the experts were recommending weren't working for me, and clearly weren't working for everyone else, then maybe I should stop listening to these experts and start using my brain.

It was a very important moment in my life. It is one of those moments that I can remember as clearly as when it occurred. I realized that all of the advice, all of the expert instruction wasn't working for anyone. In a significant way, it wasn't our fault that no one was getting thinner, but I don't mean to dump the personal responsibility onto anyone else here. **Obviously we are all responsible for ourselves**, just that we weren't ignoring the experts and that was why we were fat, but exactly the opposite, because we were following the experts, we were getting fatter. I knew I had been trying. I had been working hard, and I realized right there, that so had many, many others. These weren't stupid people, these were lawyers, accountants, doctors even. These weren't lazy people, these were driven people who had raised families, gotten degrees and earned awards.

Clearly something was wrong. This was during the low-fat lifestyle recommendation that was being suggested by everyone. Given the hype a few years earlier and all of the products on the market, it seemed as though we were all going to be thin any day now. What a disaster that turned out to be.

So, I was standing there and I realized that I had to find out what was wrong. I had been sold a bill of goods and I was damn well determined to figure out why it wasn't working. I also promised myself right there and then, that if I came up with the answers to these questions, even if just for people like me, I would share them. I believe I have come up with the answers and this is my attempt at sharing them.

As discouraging and sad as my long and inexorable slide into a cycle of weight gain has been for me, the loss of weight and regaining of myself has been equally uplifting and liberating. I feel tremendously fortunate for what I have been able to achieve over the last six years or so   I have become fit yet been able to hold onto and maybe even embrace my un-fit self. Give me a moment to explain what I mean by this.

A Little Background

After several successful steps to become fitter, the first of which I will share with you in Chapter 3, I ended up losing about 20 pounds. Along with losing the 20 pounds though I ended up with a number of successful athletes as friends. These people were very fit, ridiculously fit. They exercised at least 6 times a week, watched what they ate, didn't like junk food, drank in moderation, excelled at sport and almost never watched TV. Even today it strikes me as odd that we became friends, but I am very grateful for their friendships, not only because they helped me find this path to fitness, but moreover because they are good people and a pleasure to know.

My daughters were in preschool and kindergarten at the time, and anyone with kids knows that this is a time when you end up making a lot of new friends, whether you want to or not. I was one of those dads who was in the 'not' category. I had a bunch of good friends, I really didn't need any more and I hated the fake front that so many parents put up around other parents, myself included. You really don't know these people and you don't want judgmental parents making things difficult for your child, so for all intents and purposes it is just easier to say 'Hey' to the other parents in the morning when you drop off your kids and leave it at that. The parents you want to avoid most are the ones that pretty much live at the school and get involved in every aspect of their child's life. These are the people who you know could be trouble.

In any case, if you are married with kids you also know that your plans aren't always your plans. My wife ended up becoming friends with a very nice mother of a child in my daughter's preschool and we ended up going on an overnight trip together as two families. I remember when the two of us dads met up, there was a palpable sense of neither of us wanting to be there and although we never said it out loud, our body language was clearly shouting, "I have all the friends I need". Later that night as we were all sitting around drinking the bottle of tequila that I brought with me, we were having such a good time, that we forgot that we didn't want any more friends.

So with serendipitous events such as that, I began to make more and more new friends and they coincidentally were remarkably fit and active. I wasn't. True I didn't look fat anymore, but I was clearly overweight. I was about 25 pounds overweight. For some reason though, the fit people didn't see me as a fat person and I lived amongst them. They had some inkling that I wasn't like them, that I like to go out partying, that I loved bad foods and made bad food choices, but they sort of ignored that. It was during this time that I discovered that fit people are totally different people from us.

These people are really are nothing like the people I have known all of my life. My earlier friends did enjoy the fact that I was fat, in a schadenfreude sort of way. It was kind of ironic because I was pretty fit and good looking in high school and I lost all of that after University. In any case, though, they did have a, "there but by the grace of God go I", sort of empathy to their amusement, as they knew any one of them could start to gain weight and end up in the cycle I was in. The new friends I quickly discovered didn't like fat people at all, and really had no empathy for them. None.

The actual differences that I began to discover led me to the realization that we are totally different people, different classes of people with wholly different values. I call them the **fit people**, but this isn't a description of their weight as much as it is a description of their core identity.

What I mean by fit people isn't exactly that they are in great shape, although they are, just that they are in great shape because they are lucky enough to have as habits, desires and behaviors, those habits, desires and behaviors that will end up in fitness as an outcome. It isn't coincidence that these people find fast food repugnant. They prefer going to bed early and getting up and going for a run before the sun comes up to having another drink and ending the night at some diner eating a chili-cheeseburger. These people are nothing like us, the **un-fit people**. We have always known that their lives are less colorful and exciting than ours. We know, even as we inch our way to the grave with every deep fried onion ring, that we wouldn't change places with them, yet still, as we age and get more and more overweight and less and less a shape we are proud of, we want to find a way to not commit suicide by sedentary behavior and over-consumption, and that is where studying the fit people comes in.

Sometimes a fit person can become overweight and a non-fit person can get a great lean body, yet because I use the term to describe their core values, they haven't changed. The fit person, who may have been injured and therefore cannot exercise, is still a fit person, even when they are overweight, and the un-fit person may always have the same debilitating love for food while still being able to find ways to manage their weight, without ever becoming a fit person. In fact, this is precisely what I am hoping to teach you. Some of you might jump the fence and become a fit person altogether; it does happen, but that isn't what I am trying to teach you here.

As well, remember that fit people sometimes do gain weight, most often when injured or when pregnant. This is one of the key tricks that they play on us all. They gain weight temporarily, and then lose it as soon as they become active again. They will then claim they know what it is like to be overweight and to be one of us. They do know what it is like to be overweight, but they don't have a clue of what it is like to be one of us. These people are constantly recruited by shady nutritional supplement companies and crappy exercise device manufactures and they make us feel even more useless because we look at them and they make weight-loss look easy. It is easy, for them, but that doesn't make it easy for us.

In this book, what I am trying to do is educate you as to why fit people are fit, what core values and differences there are between them and us, and use those differences to learn how we can modify our behaviors to get lean without ever giving up the person we have enjoyed being.

Throughout this book I am going to share with you some of the unchangeable, immutable truths that all fit people share. I am going to call these the **Laws of Fit People**. I will then share with you a lesson and an action plan to make the necessary changes outlined in each chapter. Finally I will close each chapter with a description of the major differences between fit people and un-fit people in order to share with you how fundamental these differences are and let you find some additional areas where you can make life changes.

Oh, by the way, don't tell a fit person that you think that he or she is different. The most consistent thing I have found with fit people is that they think we are just like them. Only they think we are lazy and have no self control. We are slovenly pigs that can't help but chow down on Super Big Gulps and Double Cheeseburgers all day long. We are too stupid to know what foods are bad for us. They get very upset when you try to point out that the difference might be in the habits we learned as children. Our love for fatty, unhealthy foods, and salty deep fried snacks. Our need for chocolate and our inability to successfully develop an exercise plan or our poor goal setting and plan making when it comes to exercise. No, their viewpoint is is that they are hard working and smart and we aren't.

Law of fit people #1

Only change one thing at a time. Success is assured, there is no need to rush

When doing anything, especially sport, fit people always focus on only one thing. There is no rush to make massive changes. This is because success for them is assured. Think about it, they aren't going to quit. People who incorporate too many items right away are desperate. They are too rushed, they don't believe in themselves or their motivations. We, the un-fit people won't find it odd to incorporate an entirely new lifestyle for 2 frantic weeks thinking this will make us fit. It won't. Fit people will try a small change to see if they can sustain it for a lifetime. This they can do.

Lesson #1: Change

You don't want to be the frantic person any longer; in fact, you can't afford to be that person any longer. You need to pick one small element and focus on it. Make small meaningful lifelong changes. As you move forward through this book, there will be many changes that you are going to have to incorporate into your life. I don't want you to try to do them all at once. I want you to take your time with each element and focus only on that. Each chapter will tell you about how long to spend on it, so you won't have to guess if you have mastered it. As well, the instructions in each chapter are clear as to what you need to achieve before moving on.

I need you to move your focus out further than you are used to. Most short diets are frenetic bursts of energy and effort. These succeed in the short run because you work so hard, but they can't work in the long run because the same thing that makes it so compelling in the short run, won't work for the long run. What works in the long run is slow purposeful change. Change one thing at a time as you move through this book. Don't rush yourself. You future of fitness is really that easy. Keep your eyes on the prize and you will succeed.

Action Plan

1. Your action plan is to read this book cover to cover. Then follow the action plans starting with the next chapter. Do not try to make more than one change at a time. Do not rush ahead. Do not try to run a marathon next month. None of that is sustainable and that kind of thinking will get you in trouble.

2.   When you have a chance, go on twitter and search 'starting diet'. Look at all of the people lamenting that their last diet failed, but they are starting again with this new cabbage diet, or lemonade cleanse. They will be back in two weeks or a month, tweeting about starting their diet again. Hell, this could have even been you. I want you think about those people and their short term solutions while you move forward through this book. You will quickly see how foolish that attitude is and how likely it is to end in failure.

3.   Finally, I want you to start thinking of a mantra. A personal saying that you can repeat to yourself to slow yourself down. I know this sounds strange, but right now the biggest mistake you can make, the most likely thing you are going to do wrong, is push too hard too fast. In fact, even as you move along, this will more often than not be the behavior that will get you in trouble. My mantra is "This is a marathon, not a sprint". With this, I remind myself constantly that the behaviors that I need to incorporate into my life are of the slow and steady variety. Think about a long distance runner trying to sprint for the first 5 kilometers instead of pacing himself or herself. That runner would never win after giving his or her all in the beginning. That is the way I want you to think of the changes in this book. You are welcome to

use my mantra; after all, I didn't invent it or anything. I borrowed it from someone else and used it as 'mine'. Another great mantra is 'A long journey begins with one step'. Think every time you run, every time you start training that you are moving along that journey to fitness and every step is necessary and important. Every single step.

Biggest Difference #1: Relationship with Food

I would say that the largest difference that I have noticed between fit people and un-fit people is their relationships with food. I would be hard pressed to find an overweight, un-fit person who doesn't have an unhealthy relationship with food. Some people are emotional eaters, others are clearly addicted to specific unhealthy foods, yet at the core of both of these behaviors is a sensual love of eating. We love refined carbohydrates and fats. We cannot get enough of them. Because of this, we center our lives around food.

For many of us, dining out is our most constant entertainment and probably our only family face time. Food connects us with our youth and childhood where many bad food habits were established and have since become part of our traditional diets. Food is also one of the only allowable vices.

Everyone eats and everyone must eat to survive, but those of us with a less healthy relationship with food eat for its pure enjoyment. Because of this, addiction to food is so much harder to detect than addiction to drugs or alcohol. We all sit down at the table and eat. Fit people are seen at our favorite casual dining establishment too, but they don't see food the same way we do.

Fit people tend to eat for fuel. This is one of those things you can't ask them though because they prefer to think that we are all the same, but they have more willpower than we do. That isn't the case. They love vegetables and often talk about the freshness of the foods they are eating (I can't think of one time that I have heard an un-fit person talk about the freshness of a food, except referring to how long it has been out of the deep frier or under the heat lamps). Fit people don't like the fattier foods nor do they like the saltier foods. Fit people are certainly pickier eaters than the unfit, but in a totally different way. If you were to set out a range of foods on a table, everything from salads and tofu on one end to cheeseburgers and burritos at the other, you could tell the unfit people from the fit people right away. They would each gravitate to their own end of the table as they wouldn't even want the same foods.

As you move towards getting healthy but keeping your lifestyle, you will need to explore your relationship with food. Are you an emotional eater? Are you addicted to certain foods? I know for me, eating is a deep, primal pleasure. After getting married and having kids, I found that I was losing these visceral connections to life so I ended up depending on food to keep me happy. I have since added some physical activities that are healthy choices and learned how to moderate my love of eating. I certainly don't get it right every time, as I am not a fit person, but I can manage my love of food and still live life to the fullest. By being aware of your relationship with food, and hopefully over time taking steps to moderate it, following the steps in this book, you should be able to enjoy all of the aspects of life you currently do and lose weight and find some new fantastic aspects of yourself that you hadn't even imagined.

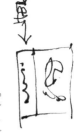

The 'You Are Not A Fit Person' Program

	PHASE 1	PHASE 2	PHASE 3	PHASE 4
Estimated Timeline	1 - 2 months	1 - 3 months	2 - 4 months	Periodic
What You Will Learn	Get a new look at the overall problem of weight loss. Understand the role of planning in your success. Make significant steps to lose weight.	Find a new way to exercise. Select a plan based upon your fitness level. Get your medical clearance out of the way. Get proper training gear.	Continue on with your fitness successes. Re-evaluate your meals and redesign them to be easy, healthy and filling. Create your fallback position.	Ramp up your fitness activity. Become strict with your eating plan.
Where To Find This Information	CHAPTER 1: The Day My World Changed; CHAPTER 2: Goal Setting and Planning; CHAPTER 3: The Low Hanging Fruit; CHAPTER 10: Obstacles	CHAPTER 4: How to Exercise Like a Fit Person; CHAPTER 10: Obstacles	CHAPTER 5: How to Eat Like a Fit Person; CHAPTER 6: Organize Yourself Like A Fit Person; CHAPTER 7: Take A Look At Yourself; CHAPTER 10: Obstacles	CHAPTER 8: Where To Go From Here; CHAPTER 9: How to Work Like A Fit Person; CHAPTER 10: Obstacles

Although the activities and behaviors recommended in You Are Not A Fit Person are not packaged up in phases specifically, they are to be followed in order. This is a rough estimate of the time involved in each portion of the recommendations and advice from within You Are Not A Fit Person. Please do not rush yourself by incorporating these habits too quickly, they are intended as habits for a lifetime.

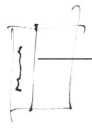

Chapter 2
Goal Setting and Planning

Setting a goal is not the main thing. It is deciding how you will go about achieving it and staying with that plan ~Tom Landry

This is the beginning of your behavior changes so that you can succeed in your dream of losing weight. This is the first significant step for you. You need to start actively participating in changing your life habits to get fit, yet maintain your essential self. Goal setting and planning is fundamental to achieving your dream of losing weight. Goal setting and planning helps you to focus your time and energy on elements that really matter. Lets face it, most people don't have enough time or energy. That is one of the leading causes of weight gain, or more correctly a leading cause of the failure to lose weight (the cause of weight gain is over consumption). Using the time you have effectively is going to be very important.

More important though, especially for fitness and nutrition, is that many of the tasks set before you are long and it is easy to lose focus and become disheartened. By setting goals, developing a plan and monitoring your progress, you can turn what used to be a long grind into a forward moving progression of successes.

Remember all of this and use it, not only for weight loss, but for everything in your life. In the action plan section we will break this down in 3 steps:

1. First we will define what a reasonable goal is and how to create it.
2. Second, we will illustrate what a logical plan is and how to develop one.
3. Third, we will examine techniques to help you achieve your goal, as this is a new skill to you and you will probably need some help in developing it.

A Little Background

Before I go on about this though, I want to share a story about when I discovered the difference between a dream and a goal and how important that difference is. About 4 years ago. I had won a trip to play in Aruba in the World Poker Tour. I was very excited and I was standing by the pool at the opening party, several days before my first day of play. I was nervous, but about half of the people there were clearly at their first major poker tournament. We all ended up chatting as the night went on and a constant discussion/comment kept coming up. In one form or another, just about everyone would say, 'My goal is to get through the first day' (it happened to be a 3 day tournament). Even then, not understanding goal setting, this struck me as an odd thing to say. My dream was to win the whole thing. Their goal was no different than my dream, only smaller. If they were to achieve their goal it wasn't because of their goal setting, because their goal was not discernibly connected to their behavior, therefore their goal setting didn't give them any plan on how to play their cards. It was simply a dream.

Later, as I was floating in the Caribbean Sea, looking at the sky, calming my mind, waiting for the tournament to begin, I thought about what my goal was. I set my goal to play an aggressive style of poker, to bet strong and try to confuse others at my table. This was something I could control, although keeping a style of play with so much money involved and so many great players at the table is actually quite difficult. I figured with so many new people at the tables in the same position, and so many wishing to not go out on the first day, a lot of people would play conservatively. I did very well at playing my game. I actually played a better game of poker because of my goal than I thought I would given my nerves. I don't know if I would otherwise have had the nerve to come over the top with an all in bet when I got a very large raise from someone trying to steal my not insubstantial blinds and me holding nothing. I shot this raise in without blinking and took his bet as he had to fold. I played many of my hands very well because I had set a goal that I knew exactly how I had to play to keep it. When I got knocked out, it was because of some terrible luck, which is part of the game of poker. And this is why you can't set goals regarding the outcome in events that involve luck as a factor.

Winning a poker tournament takes a lot of skill, but it also takes a lot of luck. Surviving a day of poker with a lot of good players isn't something you can control. It depends on getting lucky. Setting a goal to play a certain way is in your control, it helps to focus your actions and in turn helps achieve your dream. Even in events designed around luck such as poker, you still can focus on what is in your control and set logical goals. When dealing with fitness, so much more is within your control that it is much easier to set goals and develop plans that will lead to success. For it to be a goal and not a dream, you **can't depend** on aspects that you can't control.

The real problem with setting goals that you can't control is that you may have done the best you could. You may have worked really hard, but in the end none of that mattered because you couldn't have achieved your goal no matter how hard you tried. Does that sound like your last attempt to 'Lose Weight'? It described mine perfectly for years. Losing weight doesn't depend directly on you. If there was a direct correlation-a long run connection-then diets would work. Research shows that diets don't help you lose weight.

Law of fit people #2
If you have a reasonable goal, and a logical plan you can achieve that goal.

I know that sounds very basic, but really, every part of the success of your life lies in that simple sentence and I am willing to bet that most of your past failures lacked one or the other element of that law.

Remember, if you can't develop a plan to achieve it, it isn't a goal, it is a dream. In fact, that is what we are going to use as the definition of a goal. You need to be able to develop an actual plan to achieve your goal.

Lesson #2 Goals and Plans

First I will explain what makes up a reasonable goal and how to generate one. Then I will explain what a logical plan is and where to find one.

A Reasonable Goal

Losing weight is not a reasonable goal. It isn't a goal at all in fact. You may notice that earlier in this chapter and throughout the book, I refer to losing weight as a dream. Your dream in fact. That is because, for lack of a better word, that is what it is. The difference between a dream and a goal is that **a dream is a wish and a goal is a precise outcome that is within your control to achieve.**

There are 4 conditions that must be met to turn a dream into a goal. These are:

1. it is within your control to reach,
2. it is specific and measurable,
3. it allows you to check in and modify and
4. has a start and an end

Goals are things that are within your control

I want to be very clear about what I am talking about here. Many of the things we set as goals depend on others for their success. In some sense all goals depend on external forces for their success, but in a very real sense, some things are entirely in your power, and others are not. A simple example to explain this is the following two similar goals, getting an A in a class, and studying 8 hours a week for the same class. The reality is that there are many things that could affect your ability to get an A. Setting a goal that you can't control the outcome of will dramatically affect your ability to properly feedback and make improvements in your goal setting skills. As well, setting the outcome of an action as a goal rarely focuses your energy into the methods for succeeding in that goal. Currently, if you are like me when I started this journey, you don't have any discernible goal setting skills. Developing this skills takes time. Like everything you do in life, it takes time to hone these skills, but a major part of honing them is the process of feeding back.

So a goal is much more reasonable if it is entirely within your control to achieve. You have no control over your human physiology. You also have no control over our level of scientific knowledge of nutrition and exercise. We don't know exactly how most of these processes work. Setting a goal of losing weight is simply asking for heartache and failure. First, if you fail to lose weight, do you know what you did wrong? How do you improve in future? Was it because you did the diet, or was it because you didn't? Was the diet flawed, do you need to find another, or do you lack proper motivation? When are you done this goal? When you have lost 3 pounds, 5 pounds, 100 pounds? Should you set the goal as lose 10 pounds and keep it off? When is this goal done? The problems with vague goals and goals that you can't control are legion. Even if your goal was more precise and had a great time line and everything, a goal of weight loss does nothing to shape the actions that you are going to take to achieve it.

You are probably concerned that all you really want to do is lose weight, so if that isn't a goal, what are you going to do? Having a dream isn't a problem. In fact it is important and will help you to focus your goals over time. Just remember, that your dream is your dream. So the first step is to make a chart, with your dreams at the top, and then list your goals below this. **Your goals should be purposeful actions that will help you achieve your dream.** Many times you will not know what purposeful actions could be used to achieve your dream. Your first goal should almost always be the research to determine what those goals should be.

Before we set out a goal though, I want you to write down all of the baseline metrics that you can get in the chart in the back of the book. Metrics are so very, very valuable to us unfit people. We need them, we need to be able to look at them and see how far we have come. That said, there are some healthy metrics and some unhealthy ones. Do not use these metrics to keep track of your goal, though; they are useless for that purpose. The metrics are not the key to the goal. **The key to this goal is that getting fit is in your control where affecting the blood lipids or weight may not be**. Fitness is something that you can achieve. By redirecting a goal from something that we cannot control to something that is entirely in our control, we haven't made that big of a change in general, **but the change is fundamentally massive**. By changing from losing 5 pounds for example to running 5k, we have made a massive switch to what we can achieve. I have no idea how to get **you** to lose 5 pounds in general. Nobody does, but I certainly know that I can show you how to run 5 k. I know I can develop a plan for you and help you monitor your progress, see where you are having difficulties and help resolve those difficulties so that you succeed.

As we get into the exercise section, the value of this goal will become a fair bit clearer. The other fact about why this will work is that we are focusing on health. One of the reasons diets fail is that our goal is essentially a battle of vanity. Vanity is powerful in the very short term, but it will get its butt kicked in the long run. This is why we see a run on vanity goals in winter, either as a new year's resolution or as getting a beach body. By the time summer has rolled around, these vanity goals tend to be vague memories. What won't get its butt kicked is the realization that our fitness is on the line, because fitness impacts many of our daily activities, many of our daily fears, and has the added effect of also helping our vanity. I don't mean to imply that health on its own is a long term motivator; it isn't. The daily battle of yummy calories will eventually over-run the deep set desire to be healthy, but from a starting point, health beats vanity. What will win out in the end is your enjoyment for life, not your fear of death, so keep checking in on how your life goals are affecting your real dreams. That will be the best way to build goals that are sustainable and help you become the you you want to be.

A goal is Definable and Measurable

With any goal, you need to define your goal clearly and have a way to measure your progress. I know many people who 'take up running' to get fit and I know many people who fail to achieve their goal. This is because running isn't a goal. It isn't definable, it isn't measurable. Did you achieve your goal when you did your first run? Your 10th? Of course not, because there is no goal there to shape your activity. You are unable to succeed because there is no definition of success and that is one of the most important things about goal setting. **It gives you a destination to put your energy into**. It gives you a marker to measure your achievements against, it gives you the opportunity to check in and see how you are progressing, and it gives you the chance to reward yourself when you have done what you set out to do.

Having a specific and measurable goal not only makes it possible for you to achieve your goal, after all, but now you know when you have achieved it. Much more importantly, it gives you the ability to check in and see how you are doing. You won't be able to ignore your progress or lack thereof, only to find out that on the date you should be achieving your goal, you are miles off. You need to know if you are struggling well in advance so you can make modifications. This process is known as 'Checking In'.

▶ RUN 5K IN UNDER 25 MIN 3Y/6N
JUNE VETH

Checking in

You should constantly be monitoring your plan and making sure that you are following it. If you can't, you need to adjust it. If you are being lazy, you need to determine just how badly you want to succeed at your goal. Feel free to sit down with yourself and give yourself a hard talking to. Laziness is easy and endemic for us unfit people. We will always fall back to this position if we don't work at it. You need to force yourself out of this pattern. If you have a reasonable goal and a quality plan, then you need to be very hard on yourself if you aren't living up to your end of it. That said, if you have created some plans that are too difficult, you need to be willing to adjust them.

As well, be realistic with your achievements. If you aren't having the results you want or expected, you might need to adjust your expectations. You need to respond to your body and your schedule, so if you are having positive results, but not as strong as you wanted, you may need to adjust your expectations. Remember, this is a marathon, not a sprint. Take the positive improvements wherever you can and build on them.

Starting and Ending

You need to have a start time to your goal. For most of these, the start will be immediate, but for some, you may have to achieve other goals first. For example, if I want to run a 10k but I have never run before, I would set my 10k goal to start after I achieve my goal of running a 5k. Stacking up goals is a good idea and helps you to break down your larger goals into smaller, more manageable parts.

Even more importantly, your goal needs an end. Setting a goal of running 5k is a great goal, but if you don't end the sentence with, 'by x date', you have left yourself an open door to never really start your goal. If you don't ever have to complete your goal, you really never have to start either. The start and the end of a goal is part of the plan which I will be covering in more detail in the next section, but it is important to know that all goals require a timeline.

A Logical Plan

So, you have developed a reasonable goal, now you need to have a plan to achieve that goal. Imagine a goal being a flag at the top of a ladder. The plan is the rungs in that ladder. Without a plan, you cannot make it to the top and get that flag. With the plan it is a reasonable task. That really is the point of the plan. A goal on its own without a plan is no more likely to be achieved than a dream is. Sometimes dreams do come true, but it is rare enough you remember each and every one. **The plan is the number one item that fit people have that unfit people don't**. They can normally generate their own plan in their head and keep working at it. That is a skill that we will probably never have. We need to find plans that work, or if we are developing our own plan, we need to research it and write it down.

I have been testing this theory for some time now. Every time I am talking with a fit person and they tell me they have a goal, I casually ask them what their plan is. They never say, 'what do you mean by a plan' or any such thing. They know exactly what I am talking about and they tell me a straightforward plan. It is so strange how they all understand it in the same way. It is almost like a secret language.

The more time I spend around fit people and understand how they function, the more I have come to understand the importance of plans. **If there is one missing component between ourselves and fit people, it is the plan**. Next time you think about goals and dreams that you have had, think about how many of them may have failed specifically because you didn't have a plan to follow.

So, lets talk about a plan. For starters, where do you get a plan. Here is where the experts come in. Certainly on the journey in front of us, I will give you the plan. All you need to do is believe in a plan and select the right one for you in Chapter 8.

I have made these plans from instructions that I have gotten from fitness experts and they are based upon the current understandings of exercise physiology. These plans will work for you. For years we have been sold exercise routines and devices by fit people and fitness experts and for years we have purchased them. We bought these routines and devices because we thought they would make us fit. They wouldn't and they didn't. Fitness experts can't help us get fit, but they can help us develop exercise plans. Fitness experts are not trained in how un-fit people think or act. They assume that if we had a better workout, we would get fit, but this simply isn't true. Fitness experts can't help us lose weight but here is where they are worth their weight in gold. Once you have a goal, they have the expertise and knowledge that can help you create your fitness plan. They can create excellent plans to get you from your fitness level to any destination you pick. So don't buy their fitness routines and exercise devices. Instead ask them for their plans to achieve your goals. They will be delighted to help, they really do love it when us un-fit people get fit.

Action Plan

1. Write down your metrics. Visit your doctor and get your medical clearance and while you are there, get a physical, including a blood lipids screening. Write down

your weight, body fat % and your waist to hip ratio. If you are feeling very brave, strip down to your underwear and take a couple of pictures of yourself to put away and compare later. The body metrics chart is at the end of chapter 4 or you can find it on the website.

2.   Revise your goal to focus on things that are definable, measurable and entirely within your control. Walking 5k, running 5k, or doing a stair climb are examples of things that are entirely in your control. These will be explained in much more detail in Chapter 4. Set a date to start and to finish.

3.   Develop a logical plan. If you are doing any of the programs listed in this book (they can be found in chapter 4) then you have your plan. Make sure you take the plan with you to the doctor's office when you are seeking medical clearance. If you decide to do some other goal, you can find a plan on the internet, you can ask a trainer or develop one yourself.

Biggest Difference #2: Television

As I said earlier, most people don't have enough time in their day or energy to do what they want. Fit people are under these exact same pressures that we un-fit people are, so why do they stay fit and we don't?

One of the reasons that fit people manage their time better is that fit people don't value TV the way we do. They may have a favorite show or two, but they tend to be nearly pop-culture illiterate. They raise their children without TVs and feel bad for watching TV. They see it as the enemy. I am sure you know someone like this, I know a bunch, and they are all fit.

wasting time

Un-fit people love TV. It is our house guest that we never want to leave. We have invited it in and want to enjoy every minute we can with it. We spend hours in front of it, even when there is nothing on. It lulls us into a sense of feeling connected to the world. We will stay up late to watch nothing. This TV time really eats into the time we have to get fit. When people buy home exercise devices that have a slim chance of working, the number one reason that they cite for buying them is so they can workout in front of the TV. If the TV wasn't bad enough, we have the internet and computer games to sap whatever time we had left. Just one hour a day would be the difference between fitness and not. Six hours a week. Do you watch six hours of TV a week? I am willing to bet you do.

Chapter 3
The Low Hanging Fruit

All the so-called "secrets of success" will not work unless you do. ~Author Unknown

We need to make some small but meaningful changes to your life. For starters we need to change your perspective on gaining weight. You need to understand that you didn't get fat overnight. In fact, gaining weight is a long, slow process. If it wasn't so easy to gain weight for some of us it would be a long hard job and we might need a goal and plan to achieve it. You have to understand that sustainable weight gain (and I am guessing you, like me, sustained it for quite some time) and conversely sustainable weight loss is a long, slow process.

That said, what we are talking about here is not a lifestyle change. You hear that all the time from fit people. They toss it in, like it is something you can do. But think about it, I am sure you have… LIFESTYLE CHANGE. To change the style in which you have lived your entire life. Seriously. There may be some things you are willing to change to get fit, but your whole life? Not a chance. That is why we are going to approach it a little differently. We aren't changing our lifestyle. The whole notion of that reeks of the hubris of a fit person. "You are fat, I am not, so you will have to change your lifestyle so that it matches mine. After all, the jury is in, and my lifestyle clearly won." The fact is, their lifestyle didn't win, we just haven't figured out how exactly we are going to have our cake and eat it too (pun not intended, we are going to stop eating cake as eating cake is horrible for fitness. Don't kid yourself, cake should only be eaten on celebrations, even the most stubborn unfit person has to grant me this). Instead, we are going to make some small but meaningful changes here. We are going to eliminate some foods and bad habits. If you consider soft drinks a part of your lifestyle, or consider eating potato chips in front of the television as you watch your nightly TV a lifestyle choice, then this may be more difficult for you. Otherwise, this is going to be an unpleasant, but necessary step in moving towards a healthy lifestyle. The items below are quite simply the most glaring things that you may currently do, but a fit person doesn't do. These jump out at anyone who has spent any time with fit people. The good news about each and every one of these, is that once you have made the required changes, it really isn't that hard to stick with them.

A Little Background

I have always known that fast food is bad for you. So have you. What I wasn't really aware of was how bad it is for you. I had just reduced my calories (See Advanced Nutrition) to get my body fat way down. I was eating at McDonalds with my kids (I still haven't been able to cut McDonald's out of my kid's diet altogether. I am guessing my kids won't be fit people either). I ordered the tossed green salad with grilled chicken. I chose the vinaigrette, which is a Newman's Own dressing. I quite like Newman's Own dressings, but this was a low fat dressing. I hate Low Fat Vinaigrettes (or I did, but lately I have grown quite partial to them, they are very spicy). In any case, I had finished eating while my kids were having their 'Happy Meals', and I started reading the nutritional information. My standard meal at McDonalds was a Quarter

Pounder with Cheese and a Large Fries with Ketchup. This amounts to about 1000 calories. If I added in my beloved hot fudge sundae we are at 1330. That is getting close to a whole days calories (you will not lose weight as a male eating 2000 or more calories a day, unless you weigh over 200 pounds), but that wasn't news to me. What was news to me was the amount of calories in my chicken salad, which was very delicious and quite filling, (150 for the salad with Chicken, 60 for the dressing). The entire delicious lunch was a whopping 210 calories. That is about what a lunch should be (or maybe it is a little light) in calories (between 200 and 300), and with no difficulty I can order that at McDonalds. I nearly fell out of my seat. It wasn't until I realized just how bad that 1330 calories is by comparison to a healthy 300 calorie meal that I realized just how far out there fast food is. This is with a diet drink or water too. Things get out of control when you add pop or milkshakes to your meal. As well, I wouldn't be lying if I said that the quarter pounder with cheese meal never feels complete to me without chicken nuggets (yes, I am ashamed of my McDonalds eating). I am not picking on McDonalds here, all of the fast food joints are the same (and I have to tell you that salad was really, really good and fresh and healthy, still it will never be a quarter pounder with cheese. I am not saying that it will, just that it was satisfying and I was full afterwards). The fact is, if you eat burgers and other fast food on a regular basis, you are always going to be overweight. Save the calories on the fast food burgers, eat the salads and then on occasion treat yourself to an incredible restaurant burger or a reward quarter pounder with cheese.

Law of fit people #3
Always plan your food needs in advance.

Fit people have all of their food needs planned. They have healthy homemade frozen meals in the freezer. They tend to buy their staples in bulk and visit the store frequently for their vegetable and meat needs. They know what they are eating for breakfast, lunch and dinner, and they know this days or weeks in advance. Fit people have a standard grouping of go-to recipes that they use regularly. Think about how often you eat out because you don't have a meal prepared. Imagine if each time you wanted food, instead of getting fast food, you had a prepared meal. You would be quite fit.

Lesson #3: The Easiest Changes

Here are the 10 most egregious things that you may do right now. None of these changes are easy, but most of them are possible and actually not too onerous. Making these changes won't take any time out of your life.

#1. Do you take sugar in your coffee?

If you do, cut it out. I did this about 5 years ago. At first it was hard. Of all the things on this list, it was the hardest. Coffee wasn't just my friend, it was a family member. Without the sugar it didn't taste at all the same. It was waterier and not as fulfilling. It probably still is, but I could never go back to the sugar. After you quit sugar, you will find it has a very unpleasant taste. I love my coffee. It probably took a month to get over the taste difference, but now I wouldn't have sugar in my coffee if I was paid. I could switch to no sugar in my coffee, but strangely I doubt I could switch back if I had to. So, today, cut out the sugar. We are going to cut refined sugar out of our diet wherever we can and here is the start.

The goal: I will reduce the sugar in my coffee based upon some reduction scheme that I write down. After a certain set date, I will no longer have sugar in my coffee again.

#2. Do you drink Pop or Juice?

If you drink pop switch to diet pop now. Eventually we will try to reduce your diet drink intake, but right now we need to get the sugar out of your diet. About 4 years ago I switched from pop to diet pop. I found aspartame and sugar substitutes disgusting tasting. I made so much fun of people who drank diet pop, but eventually I realized that if a simple drink has 10% of daily allowable calories in it, and if I am thirsty I will drink 2 or 3 of these, then over the course of one summer I am going to get fat. As well, I realized that I couldn't just cut tasty drinks out of my diet. It filled a gap for me, and if I stopped drinking pop all together I would lose it. So, I picked up diet pop. Like the coffee thing, it was difficult at first, but shortly thereafter, I became immune to the taste of aspartame. Now sugar pops seem to have a terrible aftertaste. As for juice, it is the same as pop in almost every way. If you have the odd glass of orange juice with breakfast on the weekend, don't sweat it. If you drink lemonade all day, go diet lemonade. Think, if you are getting an additional 200 calories a day from drinks, go diet drinks, but if it is 200 calories a week, then don't worry.

The goal: Cut down on your pop and juice consumption while ramping up water or diet drinks in their place. Set a day to be pop free and stick with it.

#3. Baked goods

For the love of all that is holy, you are going to have to take a pass on baked goods. These are the most addictive of the food items. They are full of flour, sugar and butter, shortening or lard. They are terrible for you. If you can't quit these things outright, you have to start cutting down. Also, move from cakes and muffins to granola bars. Remember, muffins are bad. Really bad. They want you to think they are good, but they are just cupcakes with fruit in them. An average muffin has around 500 calories. If we imagine that 2000 calories a day is your daily allowance, than the one muffin makes up ¼ of your daily intake. It would be nearly impossible to get through a day only eating 4 muffins, and even if you did, you wouldn't be getting a well balanced diet (see chapter on nutrition). If you can't drop the baked goods all together and I know how hard this is (I have come close to totally kicking this habit, but every once in awhile I need to go to the bakery across the street--Flour, and have their Pistachio Loaf). By the way, just because it isn't baked doesn't exempt it from this list. I have a weakness for chocolate chip cookie dough. Describing it as a weakness is a bit of an understatement. I will never be able to resist cookie dough. So, although I wish cookie dough didn't count in this category because it isn't baked, it does.

The goals (there are a bunch):

#1. To get all baked goods out of your house. All of them. No more muffins, cakes (all cake variants including cheesecake), pies, cinnamon buns (and all variants), croissants, donuts, cookies, tarts, scones, loafs, etc. All out. Do this immediately (if you encounter family problems, refer to Chapter 10 : Obstacles).

#2. Do you have a baked good fix at work or during the day when you are not at home? If you go out to a bakery, donut shop, etc, or similar eatery need to find yourself a new place to grab a coffee and a baked good replacement, unless they have a replacement. The process of going out and grabbing a bite to eat might be a very important ritual to you, so we don't want to change that. What we need to do is make this ritual work for you. If the place you go to is very important to you, then can you find something that isn't a baked good or full of sugar on the menu? Do they have a fruit salad or a vegetable salad? Do they have a yogurt parfait (yogurt, fruit and granola)(careful here because yogurt parfaits can be good if they are made with low fat, no-sugar added yogurt and no sugar added fruit, otherwise they are candy served with fat). Would they add something healthy to the menu if you asked? If none of this works, put an apple or an orange or a banana in your coat and eat it on the way over (or eat 2 if that helps). Then while you are at the place, just have the coffee or water. If the place isn't important but the break is, go to a fruit store and buy a couple of apples (or whatever fruit you like) for an afternoon snack. Go for a walk and eat some of that fruit. Go to the coffee shop and get your coffee without sugar. Most coffee shops have at least one or two healthy food options, so switch to one that does if you want to keep to the coffee shops. Your goal can be to implement one of these strategies.

#3 Find substitute foods for the baked goods.

•Yogurt parfait-you can make your own, they are unbelievably refreshing.

•A Small bowl of all bran buds and granola (1/3 of a cup of all bran buds with a sprinkling of granola.

•Fruit salad.

•Activia plus all bran buds (an activia has 100 calories. That is a ridiculous amount for such a small yogurt, my wife has a similar sized yogurt with only 40 calories. The thing is I find the Activia so rich that to me it is like ice cream--don't get me wrong, I know how rich ice cream is compared to Activia, just that it makes my body feel like it is getting dessert).

•Frozen low fat yogurt with no sugar added.

These are all substitutes for baked goods. You can find others. Make sure you buy these and get them in your house.

#4. Candy Bars

Candy bars have a ridiculously high calorie density. They are so high in calories that, like muffins, they have a quarter of your daily calorie intake in one bar, without even having the marginal filling value of a muffin. That said, they are better balanced (if something so poorly balanced can be called balanced) than muffins. Don't touch the chocolate bars. Here I want to make a point. As I go through this list you are going to moan, at least inside your head, about a life without candy bars, or deep fried food (coming up in the list). You are going to focus on never eating another candy bar again, and when you are done obsessing over it, you are going to feel defeated before you even begin. Don't think this way. My brother just quit smoking and he did it after reading Alan Carr's *Quitting Smoking the Easy Way*. What Alan did, and I will try to help you with here, is he pointed out all of the bad things that are associated with smoking-many-and all of the good things-none. After you think about that you realize that quitting isn't hard, it is easy. Well it is the same for most of these foods. They do nothing for you. They aren't your friend, they are your enemy. They are literally trying to kill you. They are clogging your arteries and making you fat. They are destroying your will-power and your self-esteem. Don't think about not having these things you depend on, instead think of having the opportunity to want and desire fruits and vegetables, and healthy foods and snacks. The sugars that make these candy bars so sweet addict you to the quick carb fix. The same sugars knock your energy out of whack so you need another in an hour.

On top of not thinking of the things on this list as your friend, don't think about never having them again. Don't think of those times when you would find them nearly unavoidable. Seriously, if you are reading this part about candy bars and thinking, "Wow, Halloween is going to be difficult." you need to stop thinking that way. I will never get through halloween without eating a few chocolate bars. Don't sweat it. I ate 8 mini chocolate bars this halloween and I survived. The next day I took all of the candy that we didn't give away to kids at the door (about 40 mini chocolate bars) and I threw them away. If you can do that, then you will be just fine. Same thing with Christmas. As I write this Christmas is a week away. I am so looking forward to my Chocolate Orange and my box of Tofifee. I have these every year, and if I am around the store before Christmas in years past, I have had more than one box of each. In any case, I will eat one of each this year and if my family knows what is good for them, I will get one of each this year and not have to buy my own. I will try to make each last as long as possible, and I won't eat any candy after that, but I will indulge. At Easter I will have some chocolate as well (and when I say some I mean a lot). A reasonable amount three times a year. That is something that I could live with and I can keep an athletic body with. I certainly would never be able to give up candy bars entirely, but I know several houses with candy jars or candy drawers. I can't resist these. Being around them is very hard and I almost always give in to temptation. No matter what I try, by the end of the evening I am holding my stomach and feeling very, very weak and very disappointed in myself. These are the avoidable candy binges, not the holidays, so make sure you don't have any candy jars or drawers in your house and if you hang out at a friend's house a lot, make sure they get rid of theirs.

So, stop lamenting about what you can't have. It will be there when you need it. Remember, it really is your enemy and it is taking years off your life. If you don't get to see your child graduate from University or get married or any number of joyous things because you die of weight related diseases, remember what killed you. Finally, when you are able to control what you eat, you will be able to treat yourself and still stay fit (I will explain later in this book why it will be easier to control your behavior at a later point in your life, rather than at the beginning).

The goals(there are two):

#1. Get the candy out of your house. All of it. It will tempt you no matter how strong you are. Seriously, even after all I have achieved, and how important this is to me, I am still too weak to resist candy in the house. It calls out to me. There is no world in which I will win this battle. So, instead of losing the battle, I win the war by avoiding it. I learned this from Sun Tzu and *The Art of War.*

One successful strategy I have had with my kids, as my wife buys the kids sugar cereals, and candy and tons of other bad foods, is that we have a deal. We will look after each other. So, when I see something like a sugar cereal in our cupboard, I will call the kids over and talk about how scrumptious it is and how we can't resist it. We will laugh over how little willpower I have (and they will join in with their own stories) and then as a family we will pour it into the garbage. They do this for me when I am weak enough to bring Whoppers or a Reeses Peanut Butter Cup into the house.

I will moan and whine (and this won't be play whining) while they pour them in the garbage, but when it is done, I will sincerely thank them for looking out for me. It does sicken me to waste food (even food this non-nutritious), but that just helps prevent me from buying it the next time. I can't control what my wife is buying for my kids, unfortunately, but I can let them know that I am looking out for them and they can do the same for me. I has been strangely good for us.

#2. Have some candy alternatives. If you eat candy in the middle of the day or the end of the day and it is a ritual of yours, you are going to need a substitute. Fruit is the substitute for me. Nothing beats fruit. As you cut sugar out of your diet, you will find fruit is remarkably sweet. As well as a substitute, remind yourself of what candy is going to do to your moods and your energy levels. It will crash both of these. Sometimes a substitution hierarchy can work. For example, although a granola bar is terrible for you, it isn't a chocolate bar, so have a granola bar instead. Then, later on, you are quitting the granola bar and that is infinitely easier than quitting the sugar, chocolate and the flavour. I know it sounds odd, but it is the same principle behind using methadone to kick a heroine addiction. Sometimes addictions can be so strong, that kicking them cold turkey just isn't an option, so think of better solutions that may not be great, but may be a first step in getting to great.

#5 Add oatmeal and a protein to your breakfast.

Here I go, assuming that you eat breakfast. I never ate breakfast when I was at my fattest. I didn't eat lunch either. You have to eat breakfast. If you have never eaten breakfast in the morning, this will be hard, but the good news is that you can go straight to drinking a protein shake (see advanced nutrition for instructions on protein shakes). They are lower calorie and keep you quite full. If you have usually eaten breakfast then go right to oatmeal in the following paragraph.

Oatmeal is a great breakfast, in fact it is the only breakfast cereal I recommend. I recommend it from personal experience. The idea of eating well is to keep our calories down to a minimum while keeping our body from feeling hungry. Oatmeal does a great job of filling you up. A bowl of your standard boxed cereal with the same amount of calories will not keep you full all morning. A 1/3 cup bowl of oatmeal with some fruit will. Oatmeal is just a carbohydrate though. We need a protein too. When you eat carbohydrates only, you end up feeling hungry quite quickly. That said, certain carbs fill you up better. I eat 2 slices of deli ham, fried without any oils/butter/pam. I find fried deli meat ham to be a great substitute for bacon. It is essentially back bacon or canadian bacon (just lower fat). It is for the most part pure protein so a good balance to the oatmeal. I like frozen blueberries in my oatmeal (see the recipe in the recipe section). In any case, you can add as many fruits as you like to this breakfast. The fact is that this is a great filling breakfast that will get you all the way to lunch without the need to eat anything else. That is all we really need to ask from our breakfast.

Goals:

#1. Start eating large flake oatmeal (make sure it isn't instant, fast, quick or any other varient).

#2. Read the recipe in this book and use it. Modify it to make it work for you.

#6 Switch your bread choice

This is an easy change. Not only switch to 100% whole grains-- which has more fibre and therefore should have a lower Glycemic Index (see Nutrition-Glycemic Index for more information), but switch to weight watchers bread (or find a way to get your bread slices cut half as thin). I think the thinner bread is twice as important as the whole wheat issue.

#7 Reduce your fast food

Even making healthy choices, it is hard to lose weight eating at fast food restaurants. The temptation is just too great to order something unhealthy and it eventually grinds you down. Still there are many healthy choices you can make at fast food restaurants that are much, much healthier than your standard fare.

Below you will see a list of fast food restaurants with healthy and acceptable food choices listed for you.

TABLE 3-1: Healthy Fast Food Choices

McDonalds:

Garden Entree Salad w/ grilled chicken	Canada
Grilled Chicken Snack Wrap	Canada
Grilled Chicken Wrap (any flavour)	US
Premium Caesar Salad	US
All other Premium Salads	US
Egg McMuffin	US
Fruit 'n Yogurt Parfait	US/Canada

NOTE: Avoid the caesar and ranch dressings, try the Newman's Own Low Fat options

TABLE 3-1: Healthy Fast Food Choices

NOTE: Always choose the grilled chicken. Any other chicken that you choose will add 100 calories of fat to your meal right away.

NOTE: Breakfast is bad, try the basic Egg McMuffin with nothing else. It is too small to keep your full for very long, but as a single item it isn't too bad. If you can get them to, hold the cheese and throw away the top bun and you won't be doing too bad (same for all breakfast sandwiches for all restaurants listed below).

Burger King:

TENDERGRILL Caesar Salad	Canada
TENDERGRILL BLT Salad	Canada
English Muffin w/ Egg & Cheese	Canada

NOTE: I could not find US food data on their website

NOTE: Avoid the caesar and ranch dressings, try the Lite Italian.

Jack In the Box:

Side Salad	
Asian Chicken Salad w/Grilled Strips	US
Southwest Chicken Salad or Chicken Club Salad w/Grilled Chicken Strips	US
Chicken Fajita Pita	US
Grilled Chicken Strips	US

TABLE 3-1: Healthy Fast Food Choices

Breakfast Jack	US

NOTE: Avoid the Wonton Strips with the Asian Salad, Avoid the Croutons with any salad, and avoid the Spicy Corn Sticks with the Southwest Chicken Salad

NOTE: The Low fat balsamic is the best dressing choice by far, followed by the lite ranch and the asian sesame dressing, and the creamy southwest dressing. Do not eat the regular ranch.

NOTE: Rice bowls are never healthy, unless you don't eat any of the rice, which is such a waste.

Wendy's

Mandarin Chicken Salad and Chicken Caesar Salad	US
Southwest Taco Salad	
Chicken BLT Salad	

NOTE: Have the lowfat or vinaigrette. As well, the Ancho Chipotle Ranch Dressing is okay as well.

NOTE: Do not eat the noodles, croutons or tortilla strips. The first two salads in the list are twice as good as the two following salads.

KFC:

Green Beens	US
KFC Mean Greens	US
Corn on the Cob	US
Roasted Chicken Caesar Salad and BLT Salad	US
Toasted Wrap with Tender Roast Filet (no sauce)	US
Grilled Chicken Breast	US

TABLE 3-1: Healthy Fast Food Choices

NOTE: KFC is the only fast food restaurant that has sides of vegetables... Amazing, you can do really well here eating a grilled chicken breast and green beans.
NOTE: Grilled chicken only, and certainly, no bowls.

General Notes:

Use your head. Get as much vegetables as possible with your meal. In most fast food restaurants, this means salads.

Avoid bacon and cheese on your salad. Some restaurants allow you to hold these; ask each time. This will move your salad from not bad to good for you.

Always eat the grilled chicken, never the fried or crispy.

You can always order a grilled chicken sandwich with no bun, just chicken only. It is very small in terms of a meal, but it is all healthy

NEVER EAT FRENCH FRIES

The goal:

#1. Find alternatives to eating in fast food restaurants, such as packing your meals in advance.

#2. Memorize the list of healthy food choices at fast food restaurants and only eat those.

#8 Reduce your potato consumption (and rice)

It isn't that potatoes are so bad. They are a starch. In essence they are the ultimate storage system of energy that nature could create. To add to this, over the centuries of cultivating foods, humans have taken these potatoes and chosen to breed potatoes that are bigger and better storage devices until we have what we now eat: The russet potato. The gold standard of energy storage, the Cadillac of root vegetables. In contrast, you can think new potato or the baby potato as a more refined, boutique style of root vegetable--the Ferrari of starch storage devices.

In any case, that is bad, but still a russet potato only has 80 calories. At the end of the day, it really isn't going to take much responsibility for your weight issues. What is going to bear that weight though, is the way we eat our potatoes. We cover our baked potatoes in butter, bacon bits and sour cream. We deep fry our thin slices of potato, or bake the outsides of potatoes with cheese and bacon and then dip them in sauce. I could go on here, but it is making me hungry, so I will stop there. The truth is, there are very few ways to eat potatoes that aren't going to be obscene. If you must continue to eat potatoes, you must reduce your intake. The amount of potato you can eat is very small. Think ¼ of a baked potato with very little butter, and no bacon (I still eat bacon mind you, I am just not wasting my consumption of it by eating it as a condiment to sprinkle on everything, not that doesn't sound very delicious). Try adding vegetables to your potato and spices. This was one of the hardest things for me to do, by the way. I had no idea just how much I depended on potatoes and rice in my meals. I knew I was a meat and potatoes guy. It wasn't until I cut rice and potatoes out of my diet that I realized I didn't have any food that I didn't eat with either potatoes or rice. I still have to rethink this one all the time. Now I have meat and vegetables-no potatoes. I may have a small piece of potato or a small, small serving of rice, if I am making these for the kids, but for the most part it is all meat and vegetables.

The Goals:

#1. Buy plenty of vegetables. I strongly recommend the frozen bags of mixed vegetables, the california blend, the asian blend, and similar mixes. Find some that you really like. To quickly prepare them, you can fry them up with some soy sauce or teriyaki sauce or steam them in the microwave. As well, you can't beat fresh. Add as many as you can to your meals. You cannot overdo the vegetables.

#2. Drop french fries and potato chips from your diet entirely. These insanely good tasting food products are horrible for you. Absolute guarantees to gain weight. Seriously, don't bother doing anything in this book if you can't kick these habits. Okay, if you can't kick these habits still do everything else in the book and see about these guys later. Later on we can talk about French Fries and Potato Chips again and talk about how bad they are.

#9 Reduce your deep fried food intake

Coupling this with the reduced potato would have you eliminating potato chips and french fries. These are so bad. They simply are. If you must snack on 5 or 6 french fries from your kids happy meal, do so, but no more. Don't eat potato chips. Seriously you cannot just eat one, or two, or three....

Otherwise, chicken poppers, deep fried chicken, popcorn shrimp, and the like are all bad for you. Eat as little as you can of these items. If you would normally order a whole order of chicken strips and fries, eat one strip and 5 french fries and a bunch of vegetables. The biggest area of difficulty for deep fried food lovers is french fries, potato chips and appetizers. In the food list of casual eating places, I have included the acceptable appetizers. Choose from these instead of the deep fried.

Remember a few rules:

Crispy chicken, or breaded or buffalo all mean deep fried.

Ask for no cheese, or avoid all menu items with cheese

Ask for no bacon

As well, check out the menus and nutritional information online for your favorite restaurants. You will probably be able to find good picks there such as the ones on the list below. Finally, to give you an idea of how bad casual dining can be, check out the guiltless grill selection from Chilis restaurant. These are very healthy menu choices for casual dining and I highly recommend that you choose your dinner from this portion of the menu if you are eating, but note: **Our Guiltless Grill gives you more choices for your healthy lifestyle. All items are under 750 calories, 25 grams of fat and 8 grams of saturated fat. Served with steamed seasonal veggies and Parmesan cheese. The nutritional values are approximations and may vary.**

The healthy items are under 750 calories!! You shouldn't be eating 750 calories in a meal at any time and these are the healthy choices. Order from this part of the menu and split your meal in half. Take half home and eat it as a meal the next day. Really, I can't warn you enough to be careful when eating out at casual dining restaurants. These restaurants need to take a lot of responsibility for overall weight gain in North American.

TABLE 3-2: Healthy appetizer menu items at Casual Dining Restaurants

Applebees

Chili Lime Chicken Salad (this is a meal sized salad, so only eat half if this is your appetizer and then eat the other half as your meal)

TABLE 3-2: Healthy appetizer menu items at Casual Dining Restaurants

Apple Walnut Chicken Salad (1/2 size)

Fajitas Steak or Chicken(split these with friends, get extra vegetables-tons of vegetables- and forgo the sour cream and cheese)

Chicken Quaesadilla Grande (Split with friends)

Cajun Lime Tilapia (split with friends, no rice extra veggies)

NOTE: There are almost no appetizers that you can eat at Applebees that are actually healthy. There just aren't. You will have to be a little creative if you feel the need to have an appetizer. See if you can split a meal item as shown above with your friends.

NOTE: Avoid salads with creamy dressings, try for the vinaigrettes, as well, if you can always hold the bacon and the cheese in a salad.

Chilis

Soup and Side Salad (soup is excellent for you as long as it isn't cream based. Get the house salad with a vinaigrette and this is an excellent meal with its own built in appetizer.

Side Salad

Spicy Garlic and Lime Grilled Shrimp Salad (this is a meal sized salad, so only eat half if this is your appetizer and then eat the other half as your meal)

Quesidilla Explosion (this is a meal sized salad, so only eat half if this is your appetizer and then eat the other half as your meal)

Classic Fajita, Fajita trio or steak and portabello fajita. (split with friends)

Chicken Club Tacos or chicken tacos (split)

TABLE 3-2: Healthy appetizer menu items at Casual Dining Restaurants
NOTE: Chilis appetizers are just as vacant of good choices as any of the other causal dining estalishments. Be creative and look for things to split. NOTE: Chilis has the side salad, which with a low fat vinaigrette is an excellent appetizer choice.
Olive Garden
Minestrone Soup Salad with low fat Italian Dressing (all meals come with that huge salad bowl) NOTE: I can't recommend even entering an Olive Garden because the food looks so good, tastes as good as it looks and the servings are huge. The picture menu with the awesome specials always breaks down my willpower. That said, if you start with one of those appetizers and then order the mixed grill or the Grilled Chicken Spiedini you can escape unharmed and with a ridiculously tasty meal.

The Goals:

#1. Stop eating deep fried at home. Find a better way to cook whatever it is you are eating. Grill, bake, broil or steam it.

#2. Review the list of non-deep fried appetizers. Choose these whenever you are eating out, rather than deep fried.

#10 Stop eating in front of the TV

Make a rule for yourself. Only eat in the kitchen or dining room from now on. It is even better if you actually sit down while you are eating. Take your time, don't rush yourself. If you eat slower, use a knife and fork and eat off a plate, and you do all of this sitting down at the table, instead of eating while watching TV or sitting at your computer, you will pay a lot more attention to how much you are eating. You will also reduce the amount of time in a day that you can eat, because you aren't going to want to spend your whole day in the kitchen or dining room. For many people this will have a profound impact on your weight loss as well as be potentially quite difficult, so realistically appraise how difficult this will be for you and approach it accordingly. Think about it though; if this helps you lose weight, isn't this about the simplest thing you could do to lose weight?

Goal:

Eat sitting down in the kitchen or dining room.

Some notes on our first steps

I know that this may seem brutal to you. Depending on how many activities listed above you partake in now, it may be nearly impossible, but here is the good news. If you partake in all 11, then by cutting back on several of them, you will see significant changes in your body mass. If you only have a few to do, you won't notice as much change, but it should be easier.

As well, with nutrition, I highly recommend cutting down rather than quitting if the task feels too difficult. Write down each heading number that is a problem for you, for example #1 Sugar in my coffee and #11 Stop eating in front of the TV. Then next to each of these indicate the severity of your condition. Do you have 3 teaspoons of sugar in each cup of coffee? Do you eat chips, ice cream and cup cakes in front of the TV? Whatever it is, I want you to develop a reasonable plan for cutting down to a level of none. It is up to you to determine the rate at which you can do this, and the date you will be done, but whatever you determine to be your plan, write that down. You may go to 2 teaspoons of sugar in your coffee for 2 weeks, then 1 and a half for 2 weeks, then 1 for two weeks, then ½ for 2 weeks, and then on that date, you will be sugar free. Write all of the dates in your goal calendar. Also, don't forget to reward yourself for each achievement. These are huge changes if you can stick with them. Once you are sugar free in your coffee you will never go back. Same thing with thinner bread, oatmeal and pop. These are things that once out of your life, will be gone by choice for good. You will not want them back, even if you were given a lifetime supply.

You will probably stick with the remaining items because of what I call the Vegetarian Fallacy. Have you ever been sitting next to a vegetarian and had them shove their veggie burger in your face and say, 'You have to try this veggie burger, it tastes just like beef, I can't believe it!!' The thing is, they won't just say that once or twice, but they will keep shoving that burger in your face until you are almost willing to take a bite to get them to shut up, but seriously, it is a veggie burger, so you just put up with the ravings. As you can tell by my feelings about this, it happens to me quite often. My wife went vegetarian during our marriage, so I get the burger thing from time to time. I want to say to the vegetarian, 'Get serious, that tastes nothing like my beef burger, with cheddar cheese and apple smoked bacon. Nothing!', but I don't because that vegetarian is most often my wife and it is best not to antagonize her. The reality is, the veggie burger doesn't taste like a beef burger. I doubt if you had a thousand of these veggie burgers and a thousand meat eaters had those to compare to their beef burgers, that they would not mix it up once. So what is going on here. Why does the vegetarian honestly and so fervently believe that their burger tastes just like beef?

Is it because they have lost their minds? After all, they are vegetarians... No, it is because they have no frame of reference. The haven't had beef in a long time. By comparison to the beef they are trying to remember, this tastes really good, so it must taste like that, because it was really good and it was a burger... It is twisted logic, but it explains their honesty and their excitement. The thing is, you aren't working with a distant memory of meat, you are working with a very close memory, or if you are really lucky, you are clutching that bad boy between your grease soaked fingers right then and there. For you the difference is easy to tell.

The thing that is good about this condition, is that it works for everything. With things like amount of sugar in foods, when you start eating less, things taste sweeter. Things that before would have tasted unpleasant, will now start to taste quite sweet because you have a lower high end frame of reference. This is true for fats too. When you stop eating donuts, and cakey muffins, granola and yogurt start to feel rich and delicious.

So really, all you need to do is transition to this stage. Once you are there you will be just as happy as you were before, you will have just lowered your reference of sweet and fattening.

Action Plan

1. First things first. **Document what you eat in a week**. Make it an average week. Don't lie to make it seem that you eat less than you do, as if to justify your belief that you are being punished with unfair weight gain. This

doesn't matter. As well, don't overdo your eating during this week to make it appear that you are cutting back even more than you are when you start eating better. Just be honest. There is a good chance that you will look back on this data and appreciate that you have an honest estimate of what you ate. Use the food chart on the next page. Photocopy it seven times or download it off the net. Keep this food journal in a safe place. Make it two weeks or more if you aren't going to start your first steps at this time. More data is better.

Figure 3-1: Food Log

You Are Not A Fit Person — Food Logs

Date: DD/MM/YY

Notes about day:

Time	Food and Drink (include quantities)	Notes:

Day of the Week ______________________

try to be as precise as possible on quantities, no matter how odd this may feel. In the notes area include the location you are eating your food (where you purchased-for example, if you bought a cookie at the bakery I don't care if you ate it in the car).

2. Set your goals of reducing and eventually cutting out your bad habits. Write them down and put them in your calendar (**if you don't have one, photocopy off the sheet on the next page or print one off the internet or go buy one, NOW**. As soon as your goals are written down and concrete, continue on. After all, we didn't spend the whole last chapter learning about goals without understanding exactly how important it is to document them, monitor them, and then succeed in achieving them. Do not start the next chapter until you have put into concrete form your goals for chapter 5. See the sample goal calendar on the next page to get an idea of how to write down your goals and prepare for success. If I were to call you up today and ask you what your goal is, I want you to have an answer. Clear, conscious and written down. If I ask you what your plan is, I want you to have an answer. Clear, concise and written down. You don't have to swing for the fence here, you don't need to cut anything out right away, in fact, I don't recommend it, but you have to clearly take steps in the right direction. You really will never be fit if you don't do these first steps. I don't think it is possible. Again, you don't have to quit, just cut down.

Figure 3-2: Goal Chart

You Are Not A Fit Person   First Steps: Goal Calendar

STEP #_____ |I will _____

I am going to cut this out by: circle the date on the calendar

Month						
Sun	**Mon**	**Tue**	**Wed**	**Thu**	**Fri**	**Sat**
DD	DD	DD	DD	DD	DD	DD
DD	DD	DD	DD	DD	DD	DD
DD	DD	DD	DD	DD	DD	DD
DD	DD	DD	DD	DD	DD	DD
DD	DD	DD	DD	DD	DD	DD
DD	DD	DD	DD	DD	DD	DD

Fill in the days and the month/months in the appropriate locations.

Set your intermediate goals there as well (including when you will have cut back on certain items, or added new habits, etc.

Pin this calendar up in a place you can see it.

Look at this calendar and make sure that you can do what you have set out to do. NOW DO IT!

REWARD:

Figure 3-3: Sample Filled in Goal Chart

STEP # 1

I will CUT OUT SUGAR IN MY COFFEE!!

I am going to cut this out by: OCTOBER 06 !!

Month: SEPTEMBER/OCT.

Sun	Mon	Tue	Wed	Thu	Fri	Sat
07	08	09	10 1½ TEASPOONS	11	12	13
14 FIRST DAY	15 1 TEASPOON	16	17	18	19	20
21 1TSP	22	23	24 ½ TSP of DAY	25	26	27
28 ½ TSP	29	30	01	02	03	04
LAST 05 ½ TSP	06 FINISH		SUGAR FREE DAY	MAKE RESERVATIONS ALMOST THERE!!		

Fill in the days and the month/months in the appropriate locations.

Set your intermediate goals there as well (including when you will have cut back on certain items, or added new habits, etc.)

Pin this calendar up in a place you can see it.

Look at this calendar and make sure that you can do what you have set out to do. NOW DO IT!

REWARD: DINNER @ GOTHAM

Biggest Difference #3: Food Knowledge

We have a poor connection to the food we eat; we have no idea how much we eat and how bad most of what we eat is for us. I remember when I discovered just how nutrient rich the entrees at Olive Garden were. They are off the chart unhealthy. Many of the entrees pack in more calories than an entire day's worth of food should. I would eat an entree and enjoy the all you can eat salad and breadsticks. There are many people who would eat an appetizer and dessert as well. The problem comes when we think we have eaten well. Maybe we had a chicken dish, and chicken is good for you, right? At least we didn't go to a fast food restaurant again. Or we eat a large fries, a burger and chicken strips, thinking that the fries are the healthy part of the meal. They aren't.

Fit people figured out what was healthy long before they started providing the nutritional data. I bet it has a lot to do with their tastes, but it appears that they are completely clear on everything they put in their bodies. They go overboard and are more likely to be organic and raw eaters, concerned about everything they put in their bodies. It is bad enough having to have the willpower to resist unhealthy temptations, but it is entirely another when we think we are eating well and are wrong. If we aren't clear on what we are eating, even if you show phenomenal strength you will still gain weight.

Chapter 4
How to Exercise Like a
Fit Person

Movement is a medicine for creating change in a person's
physical, emotional, and mental states. ~Carol Welch

We all know what we should be doing: exercising and eating
healthy. I have heard it a million times and I believed it every time.
That said, I have heard a lot of very good advice in my life and
haven't acted on much of it. Not because I didn't think it was
good advice, most of the time I can recognize good advice when I
hear it. No, it was because I didn't know how to incorporate it, or
it just didn't fit with my life. Good advice is unfortunately
relatively useless as a force to move people. It is more like a seed
that can, under the right circumstances, grow to a force that can
move you.

Typically the right conditions are very much akin to fertile soil
and a sunny, well-watered location. First, are you ready for the
advice? Are you at a spot in your life where you need change and
are willing to work to make change? Second, is the advice self-
sustainable? Change is hard in life. Really hard. **Almost
everything is easier than change**. The difference between
impossible change and possible change is how self-sustainable the
change is. You can imagine the process as trying to cross a desert.
If along the way you can go from oasis to oasis, then you are likely
to make the trip, even if it is very difficult. Without the oasis you
just simply aren't going to survive.

I am pointing out that a change needs to be self sustaining to be achieved, but this isn't quite true. Odds are pretty good that you alone will need to sustain your change. Whatever it is that you are changing has to give back enough, on a regular enough basis, to keep you with it. You don't have to do it alone, and it certainly is easier when you can find people who will help you sustain your changes. For example, the Biggest Loser TV show is a classic example of others sustaining the changes for the people changing their lives. Trainers, dietitians, doctors, and a TV audience all help sustain these people's changes. You can find supports to help sustain yours as well. There is nothing wrong with outside sources--family, trainers, doctors, and coaches helping you sustain your change. This is up to you, although I will recommend areas that you may be able to find supporters in.

We have talked about goals. We have established some first steps. Some good first steps. Nothing too hard though. You should be working on those. We have learned a little about goal setting (although real learning comes with practice). All of that said, here is where the real change will be made in your life. Through exercise, we will create an external representation of the change that is going to be part of your life. Here we will have a physical struggle that will match the psychological struggle you began in the last chapter.

In this chapter we will create an exercise plan that will act like a map in the desert. This plan will sustain you. It will give you the energy and the excitement to continue on. Trust me on this as well, when you have walked through the desert and come out the other side, and can look back on your journey and take pride in how strong you are, you will know how much you can do, even though you found the journey much easier than many other tasks in the first place. It is one of those pleasant ironies of life, and there aren't many of those.

This is why we are going to start with exercise. I don't know one fit person who doesn't exercise. To be fit, you will have to exercise. As well, in the next chapter I will explain that diet is more important in the short run for weight loss, but you will learn that **exercise is much, much more important in the long run**. I had a hard time writing this chapter because I want you to know that nothing you do will be more important to your long term fitness than exercise, but I also want to keep you from getting disappointed when the exercise doesn't immediately transform into weight loss. It will be key to maintaining a lower weight.

The fact that pounds don't melt off when you exercise is unfortunate, and leads us to our biggest problem. We are convinced that we need to exercise. Fit people do it all the time and they have been telling us to, but because weight loss is slow and exercising is brutally hard, we just don't have the right motivation to do this. It doesn't work. This was my biggest obstacle in getting fit. Understanding how to exercise like a fit person. The fit people are no help here. They love exercising. They talk about how they would go crazy without it. They need to get their exercise. This is alien to me. Fortunately I have found the solution. If you will follow me on my journey of discovery, I think you, too, will have no problem learning to exercise like a fit person.

A Little Background

I had been going to the gym for years with pretty poor results before Meyrick, a friend of mine, helped me find a better way to fitness. One day, I was at the gym across town. On my way out I saw a brochure telling me to sign up for 'Climbing the Wall'. I picked one up because I had heard of this cryptic activity before and I was curious. I read the brochure and it was an event where people climbed the stairs of the tallest building in Vancouver as fast as they could to raise money for charity. This seemed remarkable to me, as stairs kill me. I got winded going up 2 or 3 floors. Here the challenge was to climb 48 stories. The thought of doing this scared me to death, but it also called to me. There was a challenge here and I didn't want to back down from this challenge.

Later that day at coffee with Meyrick, who is a remarkably fit person as well, I pulled out the pamphlet and showed it to him. He thought it was an awesome idea and he offered to help me develop a plan to get ready for the climb. There were only 5 weeks until the climb date, so I didn't have a lot of time to get ready. I believed from what I had heard that the stairmaster was a poor substitute for the real thing (not that the stairmaster isn't an excellent cardio machine, it is, it is one of the best, just that it doesn't work you muscles the same as stairs, so it shouldn't be used to train for stair climbing). In retrospect, I don't think this is the case, and I think I would have benefitted from using the stairmaster. In any case, after Meyrick helped me develop a workout plan that involved real stairs only, all I had to do was sign up and start training.... Talking to Meyrick at this time, I didn't get the importance of the plan. It made sense, I needed a plan to prevent myself from dying from a heart attack, but it didn't dawn on me that this was how fit people understood and solved problems, at least it didn't dawn on me at this point.

Three weeks later, Meyrick and I were sitting there having coffee again. I had failed to sign up for the stair climb and subsequently I hadn't done any training. Meyrick looked at me, and told me to have my running shoes and running gear on at 9:00 the following morning when we both dropped our kids off at school. I did as I was told and met Meyrick. The school our kids go to is at the bottom of a very steep hill and Meyrick made me run up it with him. I did terribly. I still remember Meyrick starting out telling me to run for 1 minute up the hill, just one minute. Soon he dropped that number down to 30 seconds seeing me struggling, and then, 15 seconds. For him to shorten the time twice in 15 seconds makes me wonder just how quickly I must have gone into a distressed looking condition. In any case, I did about 5 or 6-15 second hill repeats. I was destroyed. Meyrick seemed pretty pleased with my performance. After he had done this for me, there was no way I could fail to register for the wall climb, even with only 2 weeks to train.

I went into the office and registered right then. Little did I know the hardest part was still ahead of me. I have never tried to raise money for charity before and this event required you to raise $100 before you could take part in the climb. I felt very awkward emailing my friends and family to ask them to donate to the 'British Columbia Lung Association'. I didn't know who to ask, nor what to say. The Lung Association had set up a great website and they really made it easy to send out email requests and raise money online. This not only turned out to be relatively easy, but it turned out to be critical to my success. By letting all of my friends know that I was climbing the Wall Centre in 2 weeks, I couldn't back out, as anyone who donated would be cheated by me not doing it. I had to do it and I had to have stories about doing it as well. At cocktail events and dinners I would be asked routinely about my training, my plan, my impending heart attack (at this point, almost all conversation was about my impending, inevitable heart attack). This was all very exciting.

So, my training plan consisted of me running up and down the biggest outdoor stairs near my house, slowly and steadily increasing the intervals and the number of stairs tackled. It was at a nearby stadium. It was early March so it was cold outside, dark and dreary in the evening when I made the time to get out there. I arranged baby sitting for my kids and I spent an hour a day, whenever I could, following my written plan to the T. I seriously worried about a heart attack or worse, failure to get up the stairs altogether (at least if I died of the heart attack I wouldn't have the humiliating experience of being brought down in a stretcher and then telling everyone about it. Okay, I would be brought down in a stretcher, but thankfully, I wouldn't be around to tell everyone about it), so I followed my training plan perfectly.

When the day came, I was alone. My wife wasn't supportive of my task so she didn't bring the kids down. That was really too bad because they had cameras in the stairs connected to big screens in the main ballroom at the Wall Centre. Along with activities, balloons, music and food, it would have been a lot of fun for the kids. In any case, I also didn't feel comfortable asking anyone else to come down, so I went alone. I was so uncomfortable and out of my element. I had some connections at the hotel, so I wrangled some free valet parking (that helped) and made my way to the check in. I had raised my mandatory $100 in donations and check in was a breeze. They put this little chip on my ankle to time me. They were out of shirts but they told me they would mail me one (I am still waiting for it, by the way, if anyone from the BC Lung Association is reading this). Then I stood in line for my start. Again, I can't tell you how nervous I was. This was precisely the situation I had avoided all of my life. This felt a lot like PE class again and I hated PE class. As you got to the end of the line, close to where you started up the stairs, they had a group of people leading a warm up. I didn't want to waste what energy I had so I didn't participate (That was very stupid and wrong thinking I later learned, but the warm up looked so embarrassing, I probably wouldn't have done it even knowing that a warm up gives you energy, it doesn't sap it). I got to the very front of the line, they took my photo with a sign and then they said go.

I ran up those stairs as fast as I could. By about the 9th floor my legs were burning. Up until then, I thought I had it in the bag. Near the top of the building, my lungs were on fire (ironically), my legs were totally shot and the handrails were the only thing holding me up. When I reached the top, the smell of vomit was overpowering (I looked down and thankfully it didn't appear to be my vomit, although I was so dizzy and dazed that I couldn't tell for sure). There was very little room up on this top floor and there were people sitting on buckets with their heads between their legs, some of them post vomit, some mid-vomit. There was an ambulance crew there taking someone down in a stretcher. All of this drama made me feel so good. I grabbed a water (they had tons of them, and gatorades) and drank it down and walked a little until I cooled off. Then I hopped in a crowded and sweaty elevator and headed down to wait around in the ballroom for my results.

I did it in 10 minutes. 10 minutes of climbing up stairs. That is about 73 stairs per minute or 1.2 stairs per second. It also is below average and not very impressive. But to me that didn't matter at all. I did it. I did something that I thought would kill me. I put myself way out of my comfort zone and I really enjoyed it. I was sad that other people weren't there to join me in it, because it was a lot of fun. What I didn't know at the time though, was that I had discovered exactly how to sustain exercise in my life and enjoy it. Why I hadn't learned that this was the start of something great was because stair climbing was such a strange event, I never really equated it with exercise, but it was. It is a pretty extreme exercise in fact.

Law of fit people #4
Constantly challenge yourself in fitness by keeping track of how well you are doing and push yourself further, faster and harder.

I know a lot of unfit and overweight people who exercise, or at least try. I know people who run, who go to the gym regularly, who play golf and actually carry their clubs. The thing is, this isn't going to lead you to weight loss, certainly not if this is what you have been doing while getting fatter. How you approach exercise is at least as important as the exercise itself. You need to have a goal for your fitness that is challenging to reach and a plan to reach it. Your goal has to involve measurable improvement. You have to run further or faster, climb higher or quicker, swim more laps or in less time. If you are currently running 5k 3 times a week and 30 pounds overweight, then you are not pushing yourself. You need to run further or run faster. It really is quite simple when viewed this way and really, it is this simple. Show me any person who is constantly pushing themselves to improvement and I will show you someone who is probably fit already, but if not, certainly getting fit quickly.

Lesson #4 Event Oriented Exercise

The stair climb was how I discovered **Event Oriented Exercise**. It was a while later that I actually figured out that I had discovered it, but I know on the day I completed the stair climb that I knew the recipe to success in exercise for me. By the way, I know it doesn't appear that Meyrick had that big a role in my discovery, but had he not dragged me out on that first day, made me run up the hill, I never would have done the stair climb. That was only the beginning though. Later on the day of the climb, Meyrick called me up and asked me how I did. I told him all about it and he listened eagerly to the boring details (remember, this is a guy who competes in the world Triathlon Championships in different countries and all I had done was climb up a staircase). When the conversation was drawing to a close, after Meyrick sincerely congratulated me, he added, 'By the way, bring your running shoes and exercise gear to the kids school tomorrow morning and I will meet you outside'. I was confused. I said I had already done the stair climb. He said, 'I know, but we aren't going to let your forward momentum stop now. Now you are going to learn how to run.' That, I would say, was the moment that my life changed. Rather than being a momentary change from my normal life structure, my life structure began to change.

So, Event Oriented Exercise has three major components.

- The Event.
- The Training Plan.
- The Public Humiliation Factor.

The Event

You need to select an exercise event. I will work with you to help you select your first event. There is no shortage of events to choose from. There are walks, runs, bike rides, stair climbs, triathlons, relays, adventure races. Really, almost any fitness activity that there is has an event associated with it. The key element here is that **there has to be a race day.** There has to be a scheduled date and time for this event. I will supply a list of events on my website. So far I have done a stair climb, 2 5ks, 4 10ks (2 of these in my underwear), 1 trail run, 3 Adventure races (one of them an urban adventure race) and 3 triathlons. I loved them all.

In determining your first event you need to analyze how fit or unfit you actually are at this time. Table 4-1: Training Plan and Event Selection, on the next page, gives some guidelines on what events to choose based upon your fitness level, but in the end it is up to you. **Don't bite off more than you can chew at this point, that is probably the only mistake that you could make**. Remember to factor in how much time you will need to train. Can you make that much time? Are you sure? As well, when you consult with a doctor to determine if you are fit enough to do an event, make sure you take the exercise plan listed for the event you have chosen. As soon as you have found the type of event you want to do, start looking online for an event that matches. You may have to be flexible here depending on what is available. Many major cities have stair climbs, but if you heart was set on one and you aren't near a stair climb, then you may need to pick a different event or plan on traveling. If you aren't in a major city, or there are no events near you, than look to travel to the event. A little road trip never hurt anybody and it might be a very exciting way to introduce yourself to your first event. It may become an annual event for you and your family or friends.

Use the chart below to select what goal to set for yourself to start with. Use your best judgement as to what you can handle. Make sure to see your doctor with the training plan corresponding to your event (see the training plans at the end of this chapter). Discuss with him or her in detail what your goals are and what your obstacles may be.

Table 4-1: Training Plan and Event Selection

Age	Weight		Athletic Background	Training Plan	Event
	Male	Female			
<30	<200	<150	Active	Easy 10k	10k run
			Sedentary	Aggressive 5k	5 k run
	200 - 250	150-200	Active	Aggressive 5k	5k run
			Sedentary	Easy 5k	5k run
	250-300	200-250	All levels	Aggressive Walk	5k walk
	300+	250+	All levels	Gentle Walk	<5k walk
30 - 40	<200	<150	Active	Aggressive 5k	5 k run
			Sedentary	Aggressive 5k	5k run
	200 - 250	150-200	Active	Easy 5k	5k run
			Sedentary	Aggressive Walk	5k walk
	250+	200+	All levels	Gentle Walk	<5k walk
40 - 50	<200	<150	Active	Aggressive 5k	5k run
			Sedentary	Aggressive Walk	5k walk
	200 - 250	150-200	Active	Easy 5k	5k run
			Sedentary	Aggressive Walk	5k walk
	250+	200+	All levels	Gentle Walk	<5k walk
50+	<200	<150	Active	Easy 5k	5k run
			Sedentary	Aggressive Walk	5k walk
	200 - 250	150-200	All levels	Gentle Walk	<5k walk

When picking an event, you probably want to pick something that is about 3 months out from now. 3 months is a reasonable timeline for training. Any longer and you will lose the motivational factor that its immediacy brings. Any shorter and you may not be ready for the event. Again, this does depend on how fit you currently are and your training plan. Only you, your doctor and/or a personal trainer can determine this, but the guidelines discussed above should help.

The Training Plan

The training program is the key to success. It is the key to completion. The fit people know about fitness plans. They know how important it is to have a step by step guide to follow. To know what to do, day after day.

Meyrick and I developed our own for the stair climb. But for my next event, a 5k race, I had heard of a program called the 'Couch to 5k'. I downloaded it and was shocked by the simplicity of it. A program to run 5 kilometers (3.1 miles). You can get a copy of the program from the Couch To 5K Program link on my website. What I didn't know at the time, was that there are plans for just about everything you want to do. It is relatively easy to design these plans. The key is starting at a level that you can handle, and then building upon your work slowly but steadily (and following a logic developed over time by fitness experts), to a final goal.

I can't express enough the importance of the plan. I had tried to run earlier in the year. Running was recommended to me by a few of the trainers at my old gym. They recommended it because my schedule with the kids and work didn't leave me much time. They suggested that running would be a great way to solve that. If you have an hour, you can go running right outside your door, and you only need an hour when you are past the 5k level, before that it is simply a half an hour. So, I gave it a shot. I had heard that walk running was a good idea. My wife was apparently trying it. I thought the idea was to run as far as you can, and then walk for a few minutes, then run for a few minutes and keep doing this. Then, the next time your run, you run 1 minute longer. You keep doing this until you are running a long distance. The problem was that that method didn't work at all. I was running to exhaustion (which took an embarrassingly short amount of time), and then trying to improve. I was discouraged because running to exhaustion sometimes felt very hard, and sometimes exhaustion came sooner rather than later. It was miserable, variable, and there was no sense of moving forward in my goal of learning how to run. I also didn't have any idea of a distance in mind. That was stupid, I just didn't know it then. Whenever you are starting something, from now on, whenever you want to achieve something, turn that goal into a complete goal. You will fail more times because you don't know exactly where you are going, than you will because of failing to put the effort in. Also, consult the experts on what you want to achieve. Be specific about what it is you want to do, and listen clearly. Some times you don't know what it is you want to know. For example, if you asked a trainer what the best exercise plan would be for you to get off the couch and run a marathon later that year, there may not be a good answer to this. So listen if they tell you that you need to rephrase your question. Otherwise get the specific instructions for the fitness activity you want information about. This they know precisely how to do.

I failed because I started too hard. I failed because I wasn't steadily increasing my distance, and I failed because I didn't know where I was going. I failed because I didn't get expert help. These things won't happen to you. I have a list of plans. Please look through these plans and use them in conjunction with the chart above and your doctor's advice to set your first event goal. Make sure that you aren't trying to do anything too hard. If you want to start with a 10k, but you can't run 2 blocks, then start with the 5k. it is halfway to a 10k, so it is on the way to the larger goal.

If there isn't a plan for the goals that you want to achieve in this book, then go to the internet. There you will find a world of plans to achieve your goals. In some cases you may have to sign up to web sites or groups to access their plans. Make sure you get to look at some of the plans before you buy and make sure that the group appears legitimate.

Some Notes on Plans

As you use your plan to work towards your goal, remember that the plan isn't written in stone. You can make some modifications to it. If you are bored and feel that you can speed up your program, you can do so. That said, do not make too dramatic a modification to your program if you are relatively new to fitness. **The idea of these programs is to get your body ready as well as your mind**. The thing is, your body is more than just your muscles and lungs, which you are feeling. It includes tendons, ligaments, and connective tissues. These parts of your body are going to have to adapt to accommodate the work you are doing. Your body isn't ready to do the goal you have set, even if you feel like you could. **If you try to get fit too fast YOU WILL GET INJURED**. If you can, follow the plan.

A note about Injury Prevention

Injury prevention is a key to long term fitness. Once you start down the road to event oriented fitness you will understand the worries of injury. For starters, you probably haven't been that active up until now. You would think that resting your knees for so long, babying them, and limiting your weight bearing activities, your knees would be ready and eager to hold up for the small physical activities ahead. I was convinced of this fact when I started. Oh how wrong I was. I overworked my knees, having them break down at the end of the week I had completed both my first triathlon and my first adventure race. I had to take 3 months off and rest them. This was at the end of my first year of exercise, the year that started in March with the stair climb. By March the following year, I was starting over. I was lucky, too; I had my across the street neighbors, Jason and Siobhan, who are both doctors. I have competed in a number of events with Jason this year in fact. Jason is a fit person, or almost a fit person. Jason is married to an übur fit person--Siobhan, and being that close to a fit person of that calibre, so much has rubbed off, it has forced me to categorize him as a fit person. When he first saw what I was up to, after he saw me finish my first 5k, and my first 10k, my first adventure race and my first triathlon, he turned to his wife and said, "Seriously honey, if even Mark can do this, than I surely can". He was right of course. He is one of the most single minded people I know. He decided to join me in my first triathlon this year and he worked hard in his training and he was ready. By the way, I was flattered to hear that I was shaming a fit person into exercising. I think it was more than that, though; I was having so much fun doing these events, that I think a lot of people have wanted to join in.

So I had Jason and Siobhan to guide me through my recuperation and since then, Jason has been my injury prevention coach. What is an injury prevention coach? He/She is someone who reminds you, time and time again, to slow down, to take things easy. To stick to only 5% improvement in distance per week. My trainer always pushes to up that, always wants me at 10-20%. I always push myself, I always want to run before I walk. I need to be reminded to slow down, and that the only thing that is going to stop me is over-exertion and injury.

The reality is unfortunately a little more disappointing. You can be injured no matter what you are up to. Injury is caused most commonly from doing an exercise that is beyond your range of fitness, or from over-use or over training.

To prevent injury do not deviate from the plan that is set up for you (except to slow down if necessary). It has been designed to slowly bring your fitness level up. As well, make sure that the plan you have chosen is at your level. Do not add any other fitness to your plan, especially early on. Later we will add other fitness activities and really boost your fitness, but for right now forget that. Again, I want to remind you that this is a marathon, not a sprint.

Make sure you take a rest day every week. A day of no exercise. This doesn't mean a day of lying in bed (which is probably what you would love to hear; I know I was disappointed to hear about active rest). It is simply a day in which you are not doing any exercise per se. This day is sacrosanct. **Never break this rule.** Over training will get you. As well, get plenty of sleep while you are training. I was shocked to discover how soundly I slept on exercise days. I needed another half an hour of sleep. Your improvement comes in your sleep and rest times. That is when your muscles are rebuilding themselves stronger. This is part of the natural process of conditioning. So make sure to get plenty of rest.

During training, after my injury I iced my knees regularly after my session, as well as taking plenty of Advil. Advil is an anti-inflammatory drug. By keeping inflammation down you are less likely to injure yourself. A warning here though. By taking pain killers during exercise or before exercise, you can injure yourself and not realize it. So, do not take any pain killers or anti-inflammatories without first consulting a doctor and doing so under the guidance of a fitness expert. I had Jason, whom I regularly compete in events with and who happens to be a doctor, and I consulted he and Siobhan on all medical and exercise decisions.

Even if you select a reasonable fitness goal, and a reasonable fitness plan, injury could strike. In fact, if you are on track, injury is the only thing that will stop you. That is a pretty powerful statement. The whole weight of that statement didn't hit me until I was sitting in a hot tub after a swim. I was there with Jason and I was talking about having a goal of doing an Olympic distance triathlon

Jason has had a very realistic measure of my fitness-almost insultingly realistic, so when you said to me, "Mark, the only thing that will stop you from achieving that goal is an injury. If you exercise responsibly, and take care of your body, you will definitely complete an Olympic distance triathlon". The confidence in what he was saying shocked me and made me realize it was true. As soon as you start achieving goals that you have set for yourself that you thought were impossible just months earlier, your motivation is no longer your problem. Seriously, I had already done 2 triathlons at this time, albeit sprint distance. A year earlier I couldn't even swim (I could swim about 20m without stopping, but that was it). My motivation was and remains strong. Yours will too, as you achieve these goals.

The Public Humiliation Factor

Public humiliation? A necessary part of getting fit? Does this sound strange to you? It isn't. History has shown that you and I need everything we can draw on to get over the hurdles facing us in the fitness arena, and one of the most powerful things we can draw on is public humiliation. The only motivator stronger is fear of death. That got me training for the stair climb to be sure, but you really aren't going to fear your fitness level that severely for too long. Because of this, public humiliation is the weapon of choice.

The key to public humiliation is to make your friends and family aware of what you are trying to achieve. You and I know you have a plan to succeed, but your friends and family don't. They will just be armed with your past failures and your large body size to judge your attempt. They will be very certain of your failure. Because of this, if you fail, if you quit, you will be humiliated. You will do just about anything to avoid the humiliation. It really is that simple.

The best way to bring about this effect is to do a charity event. When doing a charity event, you are generally required to raise a certain amount of money. It is rarely less than $100 and in extreme cases it can be as high as $1000. You raise this money by contacting friends and family--through email, in person and by phone--and asking them to donate to the cause you are competing in. Pretty simple really.

There are other advantages to the charity events. If the charity is close to your heart, it can be incredibly motivating thinking about your connection to that charity as you train. It can be incredibly rewarding and cathartic as well. Even if the charity is not something you relate to, the organizers are usually very gracious and you will hear the stories of many people touched by the charity you are raising funds for, and you will know that you are contributing to a great cause.

Why event oriented fitness works

Once you set your goal and develop a plan to achieve it, you will find that your output, or work, is directly aligned to your achievements. This is one of the keys to success. When dieting or losing weight is your goal, there are very few long term positive actions that will result in weight loss. If you aren't incredibly driven (insanely so), then exercising when you don't enjoy it with the intent to lose weight, knowing that the exercise doesn't actually lower your weight for the most part, is simply not sustainable. Instead, by choosing a goal that you will enjoy achieving, and working in direct alignment to that goal, you will fundamentally understand the purpose of the work you are doing and you will directly feel and see the benefit of that work. This is what I define as a self-sustaining goal. You will continually get the reinforcement that your work is paying off. You won't have to have faith that this will pay off in some long term future. It will pay off now. By focusing on a goal that is integrally connected to your dream, a goal that is entirely within your power to achieve, you have found the oasis in the desert.

And if the knowledge that you can run further, and faster, that you can cycle longer, or climb stairs higher isn't enough to keep you going, then the feeling when you achieve your goal definitely will be. The one thing I have seen over and over, in web page testimonials, from people at finish lines, through trainers, and at every race, is the sense of overwhelming joy and accomplishment at having done something so alien, so foreign and so difficult.

It is this sense of self worth at having reached a goal that is so important to your future that will sustain you. The sense of power at driving your body to a finish line that was a lifetime away merely months earlier is intoxicating. Every time I set a goal and start working at achieving it, I mentally check in and assure myself that I won't be suckered by these feelings. I tell myself that I know I can achieve the goal, so I won't feel so emotional at the end of the race. Every time I am wrong. Every time I feel the full weight of my accomplishment. Every time I imagine what I would have been doing at that moment had I not chosen this path. Every time I re-live the sheer power of the work that I have just output and enjoy the feeling of my body as a machine. These are all very private feelings. They are all very powerful and rewarding feelings.

The irony to all of this is that running 5k doesn't appear useful at all. In fact, my unfit self would wonder why someone would do that. My negative, reactive self would think that running is only for runners. I would think that you would have to love running to want to do something like that. What I now know is that running isn't for runners alone. I still feel the pain and doubts when I start running. Every time. I have never had a runners high, and I have no idea if I ever will. That said, about half way through a training run, or a little longer in an actual run, I feel incredible. I feel relaxed and in tune with my body. When I am done I feel content, I have done all I can to achieve my goals and now the rest of the day (and my life) is mine. I feel focused and energized.

The realization that golf and running are identical was an eye opening one for me. I play golf, and love it, even though I am not very good. I can beat some of my friends and I enjoy doing that. I still know that most people on the golf course can beat me. I don't feel foolish talking about golf or buying nice clubs even though I am not very good. I know every time I go out golfing I am competing against myself. I thought golf was one of the only sports you did that in. Then I learned that running is identical. Sure I am running in races where the winner wins money. The winners might actually even be professionals, but I am not racing against them. I am racing against me and trying to beat me. It is a great addictive feeling just like golf, with the added advantage that if I maintain this activity, I will be fit, look great and probably live longer. What makes golf such a fun sport is that you are always competing with yourself, always trying to improve.

In any case, fit people have known about these good feelings from physical activity all along. They understand these feelings, but they just don't have that enormous wall in front of them to start with. They have always known what the payoff is. **They haven't had to climb the mountain of lack of inertia to find the easy payoff on the other side**. They haven't been lost in the desert so many times that they have lost faith. We have. We need more of a reason to pursue this course of action than they ever will.

The final Payoff

The final payoff for all of this hard work is the public humiliation factor as well. Sure you needed to create as strong a motivation to not back out as you could, to not quit, so as to achieve this goal. But when you do achieve this goal, the public humiliation factor becomes the public reward factor. You didn't achieve this alone, and the best part is that a whole bunch of friends and family will want to know all about your achievements. They will ask you about your event when you are done. They will want to know how YOU of all people could have done it. It is highly likely that they will feel that they were fitter than you, yet you did something that they didn't and probably couldn't. You will feel the jealousy and joy of your friends and family as you work on achieving your next goal. You can share that with them as well; now is an excellent time to get your public humiliation factor underway for your next achievement. There are at least as many, if not more, cocktail parties and social events with these same people after you have done the event, and you will enjoy every one of them even more now that you have done your event. Not only will people talk to you more (not because you are fitter; most people hate fit people. No they will talk to you because it is hard to come up with small talk normally, but you have given them the perfect opening), but you will have great stories to tell when they do. Keep the answers short and daring, fun and exciting, and always leave them wanting more.

Some of the people you know who are aware of their lack of fitness will want to know how you did it, because they will want some of those empowering feelings that you have. They will ask you questions that may not be outright requests for help, but if you are paying attention, you will take them by the hand and show them how they, too, can start down this road of personal successes, rather than the painful road of public failures that past 'diets' have been. Please, if this has worked for you and you are standing there, feeling the change in your life, than do as I did (and Meyrick before me), and share it with others.

The Next Event

As you are coming to the event day start dreaming. Hopefully you have an aggressive but doable current goal. A note here, but I always have my personal goal and my public goal when I am doing an event. My public goal is the one I stated at the beginning, like run 5k in 26 minutes or less. My private goal was to run it in under 25 minutes. I never say my private goal, but I shoot for it.

In any case, your first event may be just to finish the distance. That is great. Put down a time. When you get a time write it down. Now, improve on it. Be reasonable, but aggressive. You are going to have tremendous improvement for the first year, good improvement for the next year and then less improvement for the third year.

So, while you are coming up to your event day, start dreaming. What is your goal for 3 months away? When you finish your race I almost guarantee that you are going to want to improve on your time. You know you can. You probably should do a couple of races at this distance before moving on. You can have two goals as well. For example, another 5k later in the spring and being on a team in an adventure race later in the summer. You may select several events that cascade into each other once you have some experience at this. By year two of doing this, you will probably map out a summer of 3 or 4 events that all lead into each other.

The key here is that you need to be at least planning your next step before the end of this one. Make sure that by the time you cross that finish line you know what your next event is. Do your research and find out when the next run is, or the next event at the next distance you are doing. After the race, go and sign up. You need to keep your progress alive. You are very likely to fall back to your old position, delaying and waiting before starting again. Remember the facts about getting fit and time spent at it. For the first year, all of your fitness gains will go away quickly if you stop. For every month you take off, you will lose 3 months of progress.

So here is the weak link in your chain. Remember to spot those. Identify the areas that will stop your forward progress, and strengthen them. This quite literally is a chain of fitness you are building into the future. Know your weak links. Find solutions to them. Listen to what I say and do it exactly when it is an area of weakness for you. You will have to be painfully honest with yourself here, because we have all lied to ourselves for a long time. We have lied about how hard we do work out, how much we do actually eat, and how willing we are to make change. It is okay, everyone does it, but when you are building your new future, you can't afford these lies any longer.

Easy Walk Schedule

Week	Mon.	Tuesday	Wed.	Thursday	Fri.	Saturday	Sun.
1	Rest	Walk for 5 minutes	Rest	Walk for 5 minutes	Rest	Walk for 5 minutes	Rest
2	Rest	Walk for 10 minutes	Rest	Walk for 10 minutes	Rest	Walk for 10 minutes	Rest
3	Rest	Walk for 15 minutes	Rest	Walk for 15 minutes	Rest	Walk for 15 minutes	Long slow walk for 35 minutes
4	Rest	Walk for 20 minutes	Rest	Walk for 20 minutes	Rest	Walk briskly for 20 minutes	Long slow walk for 40 minutes
5	Rest	Walk for 20 minutes	Rest	Walk for 20 minutes	Rest	Walk briskly for 20 minutes	Long slow walk for 45 minutes
6	Rest	Walk for 25 minutes	Rest	Walk for 25 minutes	Rest	Walk briskly for 25 minutes	Long slow walk for 50 minutes
7	Rest	Walk for 25 minutes	Rest	Walk for 25 minutes	Rest	Walk briskly for 25 minutes	Long slow walk for 55 minutes
8	Rest	Walk for 30 minutes	Rest	Walk for 30 minutes	Rest	Walk briskly for 30 minutes	Long slow walk for 60 minutes
9	Rest	Walk for 30 minutes	Rest	Walk for 30 minutes	Rest	Walk briskly for 30 minutes	Long slow walk for 75 minutes
14	Rest	Walk for 35 minutes	Rest	Walk for 35 minutes	Rest	Walk briskly for 35 minutes	Long slow walk for 70 minutes
15	Rest	Walk for 35 minutes	Rest	Walk for 35 minutes	Rest	Walk briskly for 35 minutes	Long slow walk for 80 minutes
16	Rest	Walk for 40 minutes	Rest	Walk for 40 minutes	Rest	Walk briskly for 40 minutes	Long slow walk for 90 minutes

Advanced Walk Schedule

Week	Mon.	Tuesday	Wed.	Thursday	Fri.	Saturday	Sun.
1	Rest	Walk for 10 minutes	Rest	Walk for 10 minutes	Rest	Walk for 10 minutes	Rest
2	Rest	Walk for 15 minutes	Rest	Walk for 15 minutes	Rest	Walk for 15 minutes	Long slow walk for 30 minutes
3	Rest	Walk for 15 minutes	Rest	Walk for 15 minutes	Rest	Walk briskly for 15 minutes	Long slow walk for 35 minutes
4	Rest	Walk for 20 minutes	Rest	Walk for 15 minutes	Rest	Walk briskly for 15 minutes	Long slow walk for 35 minutes
5	Rest	Walk for 20 minutes	Rest	Walk for 20 minutes	Rest	Walk briskly for 20 minutes	Long slow walk for 40 minutes
6	Rest	Walk for 25 minutes	Rest	Walk for 20 minutes	Rest	Walk briskly for 20 minutes	Long slow walk for 45 minutes
7	Rest	Walk for 25 minutes	Rest	Walk for 25 minutes	Rest	Walk briskly for 25 minutes	Long slow walk for 50 minutes
8	Rest	Walk for 30 minutes	Rest	Walk for 25 minutes	Rest	Walk briskly for 25 minutes	Long slow walk for 55 minutes
9	Rest	Walk for 35 minutes	Rest	Walk for 30 minutes	Rest	Walk briskly for 30 minutes	Long slow walk for 60 minutes
10	Rest	Walk for 40 minutes	Rest	Walk for 40 minutes	Rest	Walk briskly for 40 minutes	Long slow walk for 90 minutes

5K Easy Training Schedule

Week	Mon.	Tuesday	Wed.	Thursday	Fri.	Saturday	Sun.
1	Rest	Walk for 15 minutes	Rest	Walk for 10 minutes, run for 1 minute, repeat 2 times	Rest	Walk for 5 minutes, run for 1, repeat 4 times	Rest
2	Rest	repeat 5 times: 2 minutes of walking, 1 minute of running	Rest	repeat 5 times: 2 minutes of walking, 1 minute of running	Rest	repeat 5 times: 2 minutes of walking, 1 minute of running	Rest
3	Rest	repeat 6 times: 90 seconds of walking, 60 seconds of running	Rest	repeat 6 times: 90 seconds of walking, 60 seconds of running	Rest	repeat 6 times: 90 seconds of walking, 60 seconds of running	Rest
4	Rest	repeat 7 times: 90 seconds of walking, 90 seconds of running	Rest	repeat 7 times: 90 seconds of walking, 90 seconds of running	Rest	repeat 7 times: 90 seconds of walking, 90 seconds of running	Rest
5	Rest	repeat 8 times: 90 seconds of walking, 2 minutes of running	Rest	repeat 8 times: 90 seconds of walking, 2 minutes of running	Rest	repeat 8 times: 90 seconds of walking, 2 minutes of running	Rest
6	Rest	repeat 6 times: 2 minutes of walking, 2 minutes of running	Rest	repeat 6 times: 2 minutes of walking, 2 minutes of running	Rest	repeat 6 times: 2 minutes of walking, 2 minutes of running	Rest
7	Rest	repeat 5 times: 2 minutes of walking, 3 minutes of running	Rest	repeat 5 times: 2 minutes of walking, 3 minutes of running	Rest	repeat 5 times: 2 minutes of walking, 3 minutes of running	Rest
8	Rest	repeat 4 times: 3 minutes of walking, 5 minutes of running	Rest	repeat 4 times: 3 minutes of walking, 5 minutes of running	Rest	repeat 4 times: 3 minutes of walking, 5 minutes of running	Rest
9	Rest	repeat 4 times: 2 minutes of walking, 5 minutes of running	Rest	repeat 4 times: 2 minutes of walking, 5 minutes of running	Rest	repeat 4 times: 2 minutes of walking, 5 minutes of running	Rest
10	Rest	repeat 3 times: 2 minutes of walking, 6 minutes of running	Rest	repeat 3 times: 2 minutes of walking, 6 minutes of running	Rest	repeat 3 times: 2 minutes of walking, 6 minutes of running	Rest
11	Rest	repeat 2 times: 2 minutes of walking, 10 minutes of running	Rest	repeat 2 times: 2 minutes of walking, 13 minutes of running	Rest	repeat 2 times: 3 minutes of walking, 15 minutes of running	Rest
12	Rest	run for 20 minutes	Rest	run for 22 minutes	Rest	run for 24 minutes	Rest
13	Rest	run for 24 minutes	Rest	run for 27 minutes	Rest	run for 30 minutes	Rest

5K Aggressive Training Schedule

Week	Mon.	Tuesday	Wed.	Thursday	Fri.	Saturday	Sun.
1	Rest	Walk for 15 minutes	Rest	repeat 5 times: 2 minutes of walking, 1 minute of running	Rest	repeat 6 times: 90 seconds of walking, 60 seconds of running	Rest
2	Rest	repeat 7 times: 90 seconds of walking, 90 seconds of running	Rest	repeat 8 times: 90 seconds of walking, 2 minutes of running	Rest	repeat 6 times: 2 minutes of walking, 3 minutes of running	Rest
3	Rest	repeat 5 times: 2 minutes of walking, 4 minutes of running	Rest	repeat 5 times: 2 minutes of walking, 4 minutes of running	Rest	repeat 4 times: 3 minutes of walking, 5 minutes of running	Rest
4	Rest	repeat 4 times: 3 minutes of walking, 5 minutes of running	Rest	repeat 4 times: 3 minutes of walking, 5 minutes of running	Rest	repeat 4 times: 2 minutes of walking, 6 minutes of running	Rest
5	Rest	repeat 4 times: 2 minutes of walking, 6 minutes of running	Rest	repeat 3 times: 2 minutes of walking, 8 minutes of running	Rest	repeat 4 times: 2 minutes of walking, 6 minutes of running	Rest
6	Rest	repeat 3 times: 2 minutes of walking, 8 minutes of running	Rest	2 minutes of walking, 4 minutes of running, 2 minutes of walking 8 minutes of running, 2 minutes of walking 12 minutes of running	Rest	2 minutes of walking, 12 minutes of running, 1 minute of walking 12 minutes of running	Rest
7	Rest	2 minutes of walking, 12 minutes of running, 1 minute of walking 12 minutes of running	Rest	2 minutes of walking, 18 minutes of running, 2 minutes of walking, 6 minutes of running	Rest	run for 21 minutes	Rest
8	Rest	run for 24 minutes	Rest	run for 27 minutes	Rest	run for 30 minutes	Rest

10K Training Schedule

Week	Mon.	Tuesday	Wed.	Thursday	Fri.	Saturday	Sun.
1	Rest	Run for 1 minute, walk for 2. Repeat 8 times	Rest	Run for 1 minute, walk for 2 minutes. Repeat 6 times.	Rest	Run 1 minute, walk for 2. Repeat: 7 times.	Rest
2	Rest	Run for 2 minutes, walk for 2. Repeat 7 times.	Rest	Run 1 minute, walk 2.	Rest	Run 2 minutes, walk 2.	Rest
3	Rest	Run for 3 minutes, walk for 2 minutes. Repeat 7 times.	Rest	Run for 2 minutes, walk for 2 minutes. Repeat 6 times.	Rest	Run for 2 minutes, walk for 3 minutes; repeat 6 times.	Rest
4	Rest	Run for 3 minutes, walk for 2. Repeat 6 times.	Rest	Run for 2 minutes, walk for 2 minutes. Repeat 5 times.	Rest	Run for 2 minutes, walk for 3 minutes, repeat 6 times.	Rest
5	Rest	Run for 3 minutes, walk for 1. Repeat 9 times.	Rest	Run 2 minutes, walk for 1. Repeat 8 times.	Rest	Run for 3 minutes, walk for 1. Repeat 8 times.	Rest
6	Rest	Run for 5 minutes, walk for 1. Repeat 9 times	Rest	Run for 3 minutes, walk for 1. Repeat 8 times.	Rest	Run for 3 minutes, walk for 1. Repeat 10 times.	Rest
7	Rest	Run for 10 minutes, walk for 1. Repeat 4 times.	Rest	Run for 4 minutes, walk for 1. Repeat 7 times.	Rest	Run for 5 minutes, walk for 1. Repeat 7 times.	Rest
8	Rest	Run for 10 minutes, walk for 1. Repeat 4 times.	Rest	Run for 3 minutes, walk for 1. Repeat 7 times.	Rest	Run for 5 minutes, walk for 1. Repeat 6 times.	Rest
9	Rest	Run for 10 minutes, walk for 1. Repeat 4 times.	Rest	Run for 5 minutes, walk for 1. Repeat 6 times.	Rest	Run for 10 minutes, walk for 1. Repeat 6 times.	Rest
10	Rest	Run for 10 minutes, walk for 1, run for 20 minutes, walk for 1, run for 30 minutes.	Rest	Run 10 minutes, walk 1. repeat 4 times.	Rest	Run for 20 minutes, walk for 1 minutes, run for 10 minutes.	Rest
11	Rest	Run for 40 minutes, walk for 1, run for 20 minutes.	Rest	Run 10 minutes, walk 1, repeat 4 times.	Rest	Run for 20 minutes, walk for 1 minutes, walk for 1 minute, run for 10 minutes.	Rest
12	Rest	run for 50 minutes	Rest	Run 10 minutes, walk 1, repeat 3 times.	Rest	Run for 15 minutes, run for 15 minutes, walk for 1 minute, run for 10 minutes.	Rest
13	Rest	Run for 40 minutes.	Rest	Run 10 minutes, walk 1, repeat 3 times.	Rest	Event Day	Rest

If you have already completed the 5k program, begin the 10k program at week 9.

Action Plan

1. You need to select an event using **Table 4-1: Training Plan and Event Selection.** As soon as you do, you should take your plan into your doctor and confirm that they agree that this is a good program for you and your current fitness level. Include your doctor in your fitness goals. This isn't your standard warning or legal disclaimer to visit your doctor before starting an exercise routine, but instead a recommendation that you include your health care provider in your fitness future. While you are there, if you are missing any of your starting metrics, get whatever requisition forms you need from your doctor. This includes your cholesterol and blood pressure. All doctors also have scales, so see whatever other metrics you can get such as HR, weight, fat % and waist to hip ratio.

2. Determine what date you will finish your plan based on the day you plan to start. Add a minimum of 2 weeks. Search for an event as near to you as possible that matches your needs. Sign up for this event.

3. Print out the weekly chart or use whatever calendar you currently use to stay organized. Transfer the activities from the program directly to the days you will be doing them. Make sure to write in the dates **and** times.

If you use a computer to keep track of your organization, put the times and events into your computer calendar program and set reminders. As well, write your goal in the following chart and keep it near you so you can remind yourself of what you are going to do and when you are going to do it by.

Goals:

First Event
Date Goal Set: MM/DD/YYYY
Goal:

Location:
Goal Time:

Date of Goal: MM/DD/YYYY

Second Event
Date Goal Set: MM/DD/YYYY
Goal:

Goal Time:

Date of Goal: MM/DD/YYYY

Third Event
Date Goal Set: MM/DD/YYYY
Goal:

Goal Time:

Date of Goal: MM/DD/YYYY

4.   Keep on your program. Check in constantly. If you miss a day or two, figure out why right away and solve it. Don't let it slide. As well, if you have to repeat a week or accelerate yourself a week that is fine, but don't make too many changes to your plan.

Biggest Difference #4: Exercise Inertia

We suffer from exercise inertia. We feel miserable when we begin to exercise, even thinking about exercise can bring up physical pain. They have exercise withdrawal. Even thinking about periods where they can't exercise will bring on depression.

The biggest obstacle to fitness for us unfit people is how likely we are to jam out on our exercise sessions. Has the following happened to you? We tentatively plan a workout at lunch because we really need to get to the gym today, after all, we haven't worked out all week and these workouts after work just don't seem to be getting done. At 10 minutes to lunch break something comes up. We could leave it and solve it later, but instead we push through because this shouldn't take more than 10 minutes, 15 at the tops. 30 minutes later we are done but now there is only 40 minutes left to get ready to workout, workout, get showered, back to work and eat lunch at your desk. Hmmm, that just isn't enough time for a workout, but maybe you can fit it in after work.... Strangely you feel bad right up until the time you decide to postpone the workout, then you feel good again and relax, until, that is you jam out of your evening workout, for probably reasonably legitimate reasons.

Fit people tend to get up early to exercise. This is because they enjoy it. Don't get me wrong, it hurts to exercise, but how you see the pain is part of your mindset. When you really push yourself to run a 10k, you are in pain the entire time, pushing yourself to the limits. So, fit people have this exact same physical feeling, but they enjoy the feeling that pushing their body to the limit brings.

Think about what a difference this makes in how you approach life and fitness. I have been living and following the plans and ideas in this book for over 3 years now. Every single time I go to exercise, I feel a tremendous sense of dread. My mind tries to convince me not to exercise and I feel a little under the weather. Even for the first 5 to 10 minutes of every exercise session my mind is telling me that I am done, I am spent, I shouldn't be here. Every single time that I am 15 to 20 minutes into my workout I feel great, I feel so happy to be there working hard. When I first realized this, I was astonished (I knew I had those feelings, that wasn't surprising, but what was surprising was that I had these feelings **every single time**, and I wasn't aware it was so constant). I have since used it to my advantage. Knowing beforehand that I am going to feel miserable about 15 minutes before I am going to be exercising has actually empowered me. It is like I am catching my mind trying to trick me. I remember that I will feel great 15 minutes in and I use that to drive away the bad feelings. I have no idea how to get to the state of love that fit people have with exercise, but I do know how to work around the problem of exercise inertia.

Personal Measurements:

First Measurements:		
Blood Pressure		MM/DD/YYYY
Cholesterol:	Total	MM/DD/YYYY
	LDL	
	HDL	
	Serum	
Waist To Hip:		MM/DD/YYYY
Weight:		MM/DD/YYYY
Fat %		MM/DD/YYYY
Resting HR		MM/DD/YYYY

End of Chapter 7 Measurements:		
Blood Pressure		MM/DD/YYYY
Cholesterol:	Total	MM/DD/YYYY
	LDL	
	HDL	
	Serum	
Waist To Hip:		MM/DD/YYYY
Weight:		MM/DD/YYYY
Fat %		MM/DD/YYYY
Resting HR		MM/DD/YYYY

Note: There is a page of blank measurements at the back of the book in case you would like to check your measurements more often. Feel free to photocopy these and fill them out whenever you want.

Chapter 5
Eating like a fit person

"To eat is a necessity, but to eat intelligently is an art." ~La Rochefoucauld

Nutrition, that is to say, eating properly is the biggest battle ground. Even more than exercise, eating well is always a fight. It will always be a fight. As I write this, I know I will fall down badly in the not too distant future. The key to this battle will be to know first and foremost what is good and what is bad. This will be explained in the Lesson in this chapter. You can't make good decisions when you don't know what it is you should be eating. If you listen to the food producers or the government you don't stand a chance in understanding what you should be eating. **Really, everyone is out to screw you in the food advice arena.** I know it sounds harsh, but it is true. The reason is that what we do know is so plain and boring. We know most vegetables are good for us. We know this because every study ever performed has supported this and as well we know that fit people eat a lot of vegetables. We know high calorie fast food is bad for us. We know drinks with a lot of calories are bad for us. The list of what is bad for you goes on. The thing is though, even with all of the boring stuff we do know, we don't know how to actually eat and not get fat. We don't know how to develop a realistic strategy for eating for those of use who LOVE to eat. I could write out a simple list of recipes that are calorie deficient and balanced and you will lose weight. That is easy for me to do, and not even that hard for you to follow, for the short term. The thing is though, it simply won't last.

What I am trying to give you here is something much more important. I am trying to give you a strategy for knowing what is good for you and how to eat and be full without gaining weight. You will find a strategy for eating healthy in the action plan section of this chapter.

If you are considerably overweight, more than 40 pounds, then you will lose a fair amount of weight following the strategies here. They are relatively loose. That is to say, I will tell you what you should eat, and what you should avoid. How hardcore you go is up to you. I recommend you set yourself a period of time to give hardcore a chance though. Give yourself a reasonable goal of sticking to this plan for 4 weeks or 6 weeks. Go shopping using the included shopping list. Get rid of the foods that are listed as bad here, or aren't on the good food list. Clean out your cupboards and fill them with better choices. This is the greatest pathway to success for you. Do this and you will be impressed with your weight loss. Remember what you need to do to stay fit and healthy and see how close to the desired eating you can stay.

What I am saying is that this isn't a diet in the sense of specific eating instructions for 28 days. This is a list of what is good and bad, with reasons behind it. It is basic, fundamental, and I believe very true information about how you need to eat to be fit.

A Little Background

About three years ago, my brother and I took two different routes to weight loss (this was back when that was my goal). I decided to focus on exercise and he chose diet. A note about my brother here. He is very devoted in the short term to whatever he puts his mind to. As well, he has the metabolism of a hummingbird (at least compared to me). Still, he is three years older than me, he does love his food, and he was a smoker up until recently and might have dropped dead from a heart attack--so starting with exercise was a problem for him.

I figured my exercise route would win. I knew so many fit people and every one of them exercised and I had an aggressive exercise plan. I had tried diets so many times and the three month timeline for our competition seemed too long for diet to hold out against exercise.

How wrong I was. I got creamed. I lost about 5 to 10 pounds. I gained a fair amount of muscle though, so my fat loss was larger than the 5 to 10 pounds of overall weight. I got much, much fitter. Still, my brother ate very well, although a little calorie deficient-- even for a diet, and the weight just melted off of him. When the competition was over I had to grant, exercise isn't the best way to lose weight (in the short run).

Studies are backing up this fact. I had heard that when you exercise your metabolism goes up for the whole day, so not only do you burn calories as you exercise, but you continue to burn them all day; this is called the afterburn effect. I am sure this is true, but it turns out that the calories burned all day aren't all that many. As well, I have heard that muscle burns more calories at rest than fat, but this is very misleading as well. I thought if I put on muscle I would lose weight at rest. Not so, because you are losing fat (although muscle burns more energy than fat, fat still burns energy, so as you lose it, you are losing some of your energy burning at rest). As well, it turns out that these numbers are ridiculously small anyways. So all of these little things that we are told to get really excited about, really don't amount to anything, they are just unsubstantiated claims of other diet plans designed to make you think weight loss is easy. Of course we all know that these claims are crap, because it doesn't get easier to lose weight as you get fitter. It doesn't get **any** easier, in fact it gets harder, so these theories have to be false.

The whole situation gets worse when we start measuring the calories that are burned by exercise. When I first started down this road of exercise, I worked up to running 5k in about a half an hour. I was doing this about three times a week. It was a tremendous increase in my fitness, it was a **massive** physical output for me, and I figured I must be burning thousands of calories. Not so. I was maybe burning 360 calories a run. 360! That's less than a meal.

See below for the amount of calories each of the following exercises burns per hour. The table shows the number of calories for a 150 pound person (and I don't know many of those). I was running vigorously (6 mph/10kmh) and I weighed 185 pounds.

Table 5-1: Activities versus Calories per hour

Activity:	Gentle	Vigorous	Very Vigorous	Amateur Competitive
Outdoors:				
Walking	250	350	425	
Jogging/Walking		410		
Running	500	650	775	925
Cycling	400	550	675	825
Swimming	400	550	750	
Activities:				
Golf (walking carrying clubs)		300		
Dancing		306		
Rope Jumping			825	
Gym Machines:				
Rowing Machine	235	475	575	825
Treadmill	500	650	775	925
Elliptical	350	550	680	800
Stationary Bike	375	475	725	850
Aerobics	340	475	575	675
Nothing	70			

*All figures given in calories for 1 hour, for a 150 pound individual.

There are some significant things to note about this table. First, there is a continuum of calories burned from gentle walking to competitive running. The calories burned show this. Why this is significant is that if you start walking today, if that is the most active you can be, as your fitness improves you will burn more and more calories per hour. You will become more efficient and use your time that much more efficiently. This is one of the most important principles of fitness.

The second thing to note is that essentially running (treadmill/trail), swimming, cycling, rowing machine, stationary bike, stair climbing and elliptical machine all burn about the same amount of calories per hour. These are the true exercises. I am sure I have missed a number of activities by name here, such as cross country skiing and hiking/trail running, etc. There are many more activities that burn calories at this level, so don't take my list as exhaustive, just illustrative. These activities are the golden ticket activities. When I say exercise in this book, these are the activities I am speaking about. Everything else is just working up to these activities. Once you have run for 1 hour without stopping you will have a personal standard of knowing how hard you have to work to stay fit. In the meantime, as you work up to these activities, use this chart as a ladder of goals. If you are doing an exercise that burns 350 calories per hour, move up to one at 450 and so on.

We all know that aerobics is a tremendous workout, but in the chart it doesn't compare to running (still I do think that aerobics are a golden ticket exercise). I think there is a reason for this. These tend to be classes of aerobics so they have to take in a number of fitness levels. For this reason even the most vigorous may take breaks. The breaks reduce the calorie output of an exercise massively. That is what makes running so hard, you do it for a continual period with no stopping. Every break you take reduces the calorie output of the activity per hour. As well, aerobics will have a warm up and a cool down/stretching period in every class. This is smart to do. For the run you would do the warm up before the hour run and the cool down/stretching afterwards. In the aerobics this is part of the hour. The most important thing about aerobics though is that it is a class and classes are great for fitness. There is an external time set for you to be there, the class runs an hour, there are people there to make sure you work hard and it is social. It is one of the best exercises you can do.

So back to my 5k run. It burns about 360 calories. How much food is 360 calories?

Table 5-2: Food Energy

Food	Calories
Big Mac	576
Small Bag of Chips (43g)	230
Can of coke (16 oz)	182
Starbucks Grande Latte	272
Quarter Pounder with Cheese	510
Whopper w/ cheese	760
KFC Chicken breast	360
McDonalds Medium Fries	380
Apple (152 g)	74
Quaker Chewy Granola Bar	100

A 5k run in about a half an hour is the calorie equivalent of **half** a Whopper with Cheese. It is just over half of a Big Mac or a Quarter Pounder with Cheese. It is about 1 piece of KFC chicken. It is less than a small bag of chips and a can of Coke. Just a bit more than a Grande Latte, and I drink Ventis! The good news is I could eat 5 apples... It turns out, though, that I was much hungrier from this exercise, but only burning 1000 calories a week this way. It was absurd. So, in the short run, exercise just doesn't do as much for your weight loss as you would want.

Still, it is so much easier to stick with exercise than a diet and to lose weight without increasing your physical output you need to crash diet. You need to eat remarkably small amounts of food. For almost everyone this is not sustainable. As soon as you are exercising though, the changes to your diet have profound, significant and lifelong effects. As well, by losing weight, your goals of working harder and faster are easier to reach so you are more motivated to achieve them. This really is a case of there being a tremendous synergy between exercise and eating better. Each of them helps the other and both of them help you get fit.

My brother ate very well during his diet. Other than the fact that it was a little calorie deficient, it really wasn't a diet. It was a healthy eating plan. I learned a lot from him during this time and we spent hours talking about what was healthy eating and the easiest ways to fit it into our lives. I am indebted to him for many of the ideas in this chapter and for being a sounding board throughout this whole process. And by the way, he may have beaten me in the bet, but since then the long run has been very very good to me.

Law of fit people #5
Eat vegetables like they are candy.

This is a no brainer. We all have seen this. Fit people love their vegetables. The way to make this work for you though is to incorporate the vegetables that you do like into more of your meals and get rid of the starches. As I said earlier, starches (potatoes) aren't vegetables so never again think of them as vegetables. Also, any processed vegetables such as corn in butter sauce or tempura carrots are not a vegetable.

Start with the vegetables you know and love. There have to be a few. Make sure you eat them in every meal. Corn is on almost everybody's list. Carrots are well liked and most people can eat iceburg lettuce. If this is all you have, start with that. I found that eating pizza with green peppers and onions on it opened up a love of those vegetables for me. I also love them in a fajita. I love pea pods, onions, broccoli, cauliflower, carrots and sprouts in a stir fry. There is a recipe in the back for several stir fries. If you like the vegetables in these meals keep eating them. Try some variations based on them. Find other similar recipes. The more vegetables you eat the more full you will be while eating fewer overall calories. This is the holy grail for living your lifestyle and being fit.

Finally, I have found that cutting the pieces of vegetable tremendously small really helps. The best greek salad I ever had had tiny minced pieces of vegetable in it. It was incredible. When you are eating raw vegetables use a vinaigrette based dip as well, never a ranch style dip.

Lesson #5 Nutrition 101

So, without further ado, here is what you have to do to eat like a fit person. There are essentially 3 factors, in my opinion, that you need to take into account when trying to eat like a fit person (and one factor for drinking like a fit person) and these are:

- Calorie Density
- Fibre and reduced refined Carbohydrates
- Balance of Carbohydrates, Fats and Proteins.
- Additionally, you can use Water to your advantage.

I don't think fit people ever think of these things, they just have the right mix, but once again, you are not a fit person. After all, a fit person doesn't plan on eating that cake at the birthday party that you are taking your child to so that you actually stay at the kids party for 2 hours even though you could leave and get some time to yourself (yes I have done this, more than once). A fit person has the ability to say no to those barbecue potato chips on the table, in fact not only do they have the ability, they don't even hear the siren song of those wonderfully deep fried greasy little wafers of goodness. Fit people like water and think that is the only liquid that they need. So, we need to be armed with some simple knowledge to eat like a fit person. Follow these rules and you will be almost undetectable from a fit person (except of course for the far away look in your eyes that you have as the fit people discuss how disgusting french fries are, as you are clearly ranking the french fries in your head from all of the fast food restaurants on a scale of overall deliciousness, saltiness, crispiness and a dozen other values, all the while wondering how these people can use a blanket word like french fries to encompass all of the different preparations, as if saying red captures the depth of richness of a brilliant sunset). Note, that I have broken Fibre and Reducing refined carbohydrates into their own category, when in fact they are a subgroup of the balanced macro-nutrient category. The reason I have done this is that they are a very important subcategory. The balance of macro-nutrients is important in your diet, but even that isn't as important as cutting out refined carbohydrates and eating more fibre. I will explain this all below in any case.

Calorie Density

Probably the most important concept in nutrition is the concept of calorie density. This subject is very common sense and that is probably why it doesn't typically get the mention that it deserves.

Some foods have more calories per gram (or per weight or mass or density) than others. Some foods are nutrient rich, others are not. **To calculate a food's calorie density just take the number of calories in a food and divide it by its weight in grams.** Simple enough. But what does this tell us and and why is it important?

Figure 5-1: Calculating Calorie Density from a Nutrition

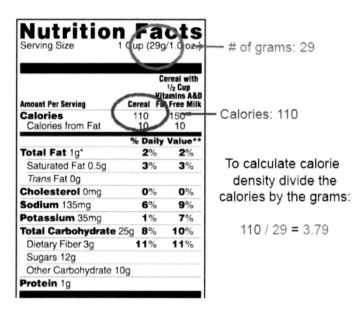

Label

There are many reasons why we eat, for some of us it is a treat we give ourselves, for others emotional reasons, for others it is boredom or habit, and still for others it is an addiction (for me it is all of the above). We talked about this in the previous section. Discovering why we eat is very important in breaking our unhealthy link with food. That said, why we eat is a different problem than why eating healthy, or reducing our intake, fails.

Many of us fear dieting because we know we will be hungry (or we fail to stick to our diet's plans because after eating our allotted calories we aren't full). This is why monitoring calories and limiting our intake doesn't work. We can't stick to eating a half a chocolate bar and a 4 chicken wings for our daily food intake, yet, if we ate these foods, we wouldn't be able to eat anything else all day. That is because these are extremely calorie dense foods.

Have you ever noticed that you rarely see fit people eating in McDonalds? How when you ask them about fast food, they scrunch up their faces and appear to be repulsed by a cheeseburger? How about what they eat. They are always eating vegetables, and whole grains, and chick peas... They are never eating potato chips and hot wings. They are also never counting calories. This is because they have internalized what I am recommending here. A cheeseburger has a very significant calorie density, by the way.

For weight loss, we are simply going to limit our high calorie density foods and go crazy eating as much low calorie density foods as we want. We will stay full all the time. This is extremely important to weight loss because your body is your biggest enemy in weight loss. You are in a pitched battle with your body as soon as you try to get fit. Your body doesn't care about fitness, not at all. It has been optimized over generations and generations to get you to breading age, without dying of starvation in times of scarcity, and then just 12 years longer. Long enough to raise your offspring to have the same chance for survival as you. Most of the people walking the planet right now, have your same unbelievable optimized system of survival. Store all excess calories in the body as fat for times of scarcity. Then at times of scarcity use the fat reserves to provide energy for survival.

And if it were only that simple, but it isn't; the body is much more resilient and brilliant than that. In addition to burning fat, the body also slows down your metabolism (Basal Metabolic Rate) to conserve energy. After all, there isn't much food around, you had better rest and sleep until there is a more plentiful time. This forces your body to use much less energy, so as you are reducing your calories, your body is matching your move in reducing your use of those calories. This would be demonic enough, but the body goes one step further. It remembers that times are variable, so when you encounter food again (stop your diet), the body makes a note to store more and more, because you survived that last nearly deadly time thanks to its defensive mechanisms. So, as soon as you stop eating healthy, your body jumps on those calories and stores them, and you become larger and more susceptible to a host of health problems.

All of this is why you cannot let yourself get hungry. When your body is telling you it is hungry and you aren't doing anything about it, you are signaling your body that there isn't enough food around and it is getting ready to bring in measures to counter what you are doing. That is also why we began with an exercise program. If you body thinks that it can lower your metabolism, it will think again as you continue to output energy for physical activity. So, the following chart has a sampling of the calorie density of foods, in descending order from the highest density (an unhealthy choice) down to the lowest density (eat these whenever you want).

You will have noticed that vegetables are the healthiest choices and I recommend eating a ton of them with whatever meal you are eating. If 6 tips of asparagus only contain 30 calories(a CD of .22), how much asparagus could you eat in one sitting? Seriously, to get a 400 calorie meal you would have to eat 80 asparagus tips!! Not that I am recommending doing that, as you would get no protein in your meal, and proteins may help trigger your sense of fullness. What you need to do is balance your meal (see Balance Carbs, Proteins and Fats). I am also not recommending it because just eating vegetables won't make you feel full, you won't enjoy it and it won't stick. But by putting more vegetables in foods you like, you will be able to enjoy the foods you like and get your overall calorie density down. One of my favorite recipes for healthy meals is the 'hot sauce stir fry'. You can find it in the recipe section. I first had something like this at a restaurant chain. As soon as I started eating healthier it dawned on me that I could make this at home, use tons of vegetables and feed my hot sauce/chicken wing habit. It works so well and the vegetables absorb so much more of the hot sauce than the meat, they actually become the stars of the meal.

I never used to like vegetables. I had to force vegetables down my throat until I began to not hate them, and then, like them and now love them. That is what I am recommending for you. Obviously you aren't a huge vegetable lover. If you were, you wouldn't be reading this book! So, I really don't want to hear whines of 'I hate vegetables'. We all do, that is why we are in the spot we are in, that is also why McDonalds doesn't sell a burger with a side of asparagus. That said, eat them with your loved meats and sauces. Choke them down. Always finish your meal with a bite of your favorite item on the plate, and pretty soon, you will love the veggies you eat. I started enjoying cooked onions and peppers in my fajita and cooked tomatoes, onions and peppers in my shish kabobs. Now I love all of those raw in greek salads. By eating foods I loved (meats) that are cooked with vegetables, I soon acquired the taste for vegetables. Try this, there is a stir fry and a shish kabob recipe in the back. I love broccoli and cauliflower in stir fries because they absorb all of the flavors of the meat.

As well as vegetables, fruits like apples, oranges, and bananas, make excellent snacks. If you hate fruits, I feel for you, but I will tell you to embrace the fruit if you are seriously thinking of living to a ripe old age. It is your choice though.

Once you can eat healthy and not be hungry, then the decision to stay away from the addictive sugars and starches is a decision you will have the power to make. You will no longer feel terrible for making bad decisions over and over. Yes, you will probably never have the luxury of finding salt and vinegar chips disgusting, or chicken fingers and dips a deep fried nightmare. Oh no, on the contrary, you have tasted from the forbidden fruit. So you will never be a fit person, but you will have every opportunity to eat like one, and in turn, you will have every opportunity to live to the most possible of your days, healthy and full of energy.

Instructions for using **Table 5-3: Calorie Densities of Common Foods**:

avoid items in the black square (with a CD above 2.0)
If you eat them remember you are eating something very unhealthy and eat as little as you can. For butter and oils again, use them as sparingly as you can with meals.

eat items in the grey squares in moderation (with a CD between 1.0 and 2.0)
Eat about 4 oz of these at a sitting with as much of the items in green as you want.

enjoy as many of the items in the white squares (a CD below 1.0)
When calculating for yourself if the food has a calorie density above 2 don't eat it. Between 1 and 2 eat only 4 oz at a sitting and 1 and below, eat away.

Table 5-3: Calorie Densities of Common Foods	
Food Product	Calorie Density
Salad or cooking oil	8.80
Butter or margarine, stick	7.20
Mayonnaise, regular	7.20
Almonds	5.90
Peanuts or peanut butter	5.90

continued...

Table 5-3: Calorie Densities of Common Foods

Food	Calorie Density
Lays Flamin' Hot Chips	5.71
Cashew Nuts	5.50
Milk chocolate bar	5.40
Potato chips or corn chips	5.40
Lays Classic Chips	5.36
Peanut Butter Cups	5.15
Bacon	5.00
Cheddar cheese	4.80
Butterfinger	4.76
Snickers	4.67
Chocolate chip cookies	4.60
Chocolate Chip Muffin	4.50
Brownie	4.40
Carrot cake with cream cheese frosting	4.40
Pecan pie	4.20
Croissant	4.10
Glazed or plain doughnut	4.10
Onion rings	4.10
Baked potato chips	3.90
Hard pretzels	3.90
Rice Cakes	3.80
Chocolate cake with frosting	3.70
Italian dressing, full-fat	3.60
Sarah Lee Mini-Blueberry Muffin	3.50
Aunt Jemimah Original Pancake Mix	3.50
Mayonnaise, light	3.30
Cheesecake	3.25
French fries	3.20
Starbucks Morning Sunrise Muffin	3.00
Raisins	3.00
Kalamata Olives	3.00
Blueberry muffin	2.90

Table 5-3: Calorie Densities of Common Foods	
Cheese pizza	2.90
Plain bagel	2.80
Feta Cheese	2.75
McDonald's Quarter Pounder w/ Cheese	2.71
Apple pie	2.70
Lean ground beef	2.70
Bread	2.60
Hamburger Bun	2.55
Premium ice cream	2.50
Chicken Wings	2.46
Chicken Thigh	2.32
Bacon Double Cheeseburger	2.31
Tenderloin (Filet Mignon)	2.10
Lean Pork Chop (no bone)	1.92
Chicken Breast (w/skin)	1.82
Sirloin Steak	1.78
Chicken Breast (no skin)	1.65
White Rice	1.30
Turkey Breast	1.09
Yogurt (full fat sweetened with sugar)	1.00
Banana	0.88
Plain, nonfat yogurt	0.59
Blueberries	0.56
Fruit yogurt, fat-free, artificially sweetened	0.53
Apple	0.52
Italian dressing, fat-free	0.47
Orange	0.47
Carrots	0.43
Peach	0.43
Winter squash	0.39
Cantaloupe	0.35
Watermelon	0.32

Table 5-3: Calorie Densities of Common Foods	
Grapefruit	0.30
Strawberries	0.30
Vegetable soup	0.30
Broccoli	0.28
Asparagus	0.24
Tomato	0.21
Lettuce	0.18
Celery	0.16
Chicken broth	0.16
Cucumber	0.13

(using a ↓ plate)

There is a great website that deals visually with the concept of calorie density. It can be found on the website under Calorie Density Images. You can visually see why calorie density is so important. Whatever you do, don't go through this list thinking of what you can eat and how much of each item. Instead just notice how full that bowl is with the healthier items and as you move down, how empty the bowl becomes. That is the concept. Understand it and use it day in and day out. This process works in the long term, so stick with it and incorporate it all the time.

Refined Carbohydrates and Fibre

My first introduction to the whole idea behind refined carbohydrates being bad came from my Uncle Wayne. Uncle Wayne isn't a fit person (he definitely has known many fit people and has kept his ear to the ground in this area more than I ever had at this point), but he has stayed fit all of his life. He is clearly one of those people who has battled with weight gain and fitness his whole life and has been on the winning end. That is why, when I was quite obese and munching on rice cakes, visiting with my parents at their house one day, I had a breakthrough learning moment. I was commenting that I was steps away from good health as my wife had suggested that I eat these rice cakes as part of my low calorie diet. I can still remember the look on Wayne's face as I munched on those tasteless cardboard wafers. It was a mix of revulsion and horror at how misinformed I was.

Uncle Wayne is one of those generally quiet, but very brilliant people, who rarely sticks his nose into anyone's business. Instead, he quietly offers funny comments and clever thoughts for you to mull over later--but nothing ever cutting or biting. The things he says tend to stick too. This was what I was left with after that day. He told me a little about studies with diabetics on certain foods that elicit an insulin response. Insulin in the blood is responsible for the body storing fats. I realized that there was a lot I didn't know about food. That all foods weren't equal. I am rigidly logical, so the whole notion of calories in – calories out equals weight gain or loss, the mantra of the entire fitness world at that time (and not surprisingly, to this day) seemed to be an insurmountable logical hurdle. Yet, here it was. A complexity to dieting I had never imagined. Not all calories are created equal. I had been hearing this with fats for awhile, but that logic failed me (I won't expand on this here, but if you were around to witness the low fat diet recommendations that every government agency supported and eschewed, you will know what I am talking about). This logic was much, much better. There is other pathways of interaction with food, and one of them is hormonal. This had been discovered by Dr J. A. Jenkins from the University of Toronto, and published in March edition of the American Journal of Clinical Nutrition, 1981. Why Dr. Jenkins has not received the Nobel Prize in Medicine by now is anyone's guess. In any case, work from many researchers showed that some foods made up of complex carbohydrates (breads, cereals, potatoes) produce a hormonal response of production of insulin in the blood stream as large as or larger than the response produced by straight sugar. Why this is a problem for us is:

- insulin stimulates the cells of the body to take up glucose, so that they have the energy to do their work
- insulin allows extra sugar to be stored as energy for future use. It can be stored in the liver, in the form of glycogen, or deposited in fat cells
- The insulin released in response to a meal is just the right amount to keep the blood sugar from going too high. The pancreas secretes less insulin into the blood after most of the nutrients from the meal have been taken up by the cells, and the blood glucose levels once again approach "fasting" (pre-meal) levels.

So, insulin allows extra sugar to be stored as fat. Without insulin, you couldn't store extra sugar as fat at all. In fact, without insulin, you would burn fats for energy rather than the sugars in your blood. This is how the 'Low Carb Diets' such as the Atkins Diet work. It seems incredible that these diets that consist of eating as much fats and proteins as you want can work, but they do. They work because of the activity of insulin. Incredibly, Dr. Atkins published his work in 1972, 9 years before Dr Jenkins showed the world just how reactive complex carbohydrates were with your insulin production.

I have had many people tell me about their experiences with these low carb diets and every single one of them has said that they lost a lot of weight while they were on the diet, but each and every one of them gained the weight back afterwards and then some. For almost everyone, living on this diet is just impossible. We enjoy drinking (carbohydrates), bread (carbohydrates), and fruits and vegetables (carbohydrates) way too much. There is a lot of controversy over these kinds of diets, (as there is, to be fair, over just about every other), but the health or safety of these diets isn't an issue for us at all right now.

The issue for us is that this is a short term eating choice for almost everyone alive, and as such, we will have to toss it out as an option. I want to be clear here, all current research points to short term diets reducing your ability to lose weight in the future and increasing your body weight as soon as you stop. According to Dr. Traci Mann, a social psychologist at the University of California in Los Angeles. who led a team of researchers who examined some 30 long-term studies of diets, the results of which appeared April 2007 in American Psychologist, the journal of the American Psychological Association.

"What happens to people on diets in the long run?" Mann asked. "Would they have been better off not to go on a diet at all? We decided to dig up and analyze every study that followed people on diets for two to five years. We concluded most of them would have been better off not going on the diet at all. Their weight would be pretty much the same, and their bodies would not suffer the wear and tear from losing weight and gaining it all back."

So, enough said about this diet, other than the fact that I have never seen a fit person live this way, not even close.

Understanding that there was an hormonal pathway that determined how much energy was stored and how much wasn't led me to Dr. Barry Sears. I picked up a copy of The Zone Diet, and my rational mind loved it. It is the gold standard for understanding the relationship between Carbohydrates, Proteins and Fats, but what really caught my attention was his statement that some people are more reactive to carbohydrates than others. Some people produce more insulin in response to the same amount of carbohydrate. He didn't have a study to back him on this, he just suggested that you look in a mirror to see your level of reaction. If you are pear shaped, you are highly reactive. This appealed to me right away because I knew some people could eat more food than I could and they didn't gain weight, and they would look down on me for being fat. This caused me endless amounts of grief and anger and probably got in the way of my fitness more than I wanted to admit.

Here, Dr. Sears is saying that certain people may have a GI Index of white bread that is much, much higher than someone else. Interestingly enough, studies are now proving this point:

SUGAMENT.

Using glucose as the control food, previous studies indicate that white bread has a glycemic index of about 70," says Lichtenstein, who is also the Gershoff professor of nutrition science and policy at the Friedman School of Nutrition Science and Policy at Tufts. "In our study the combined average was 71, virtually identical to the published value. However, quite strikingly, individual values ranged from 44 to 132. What is critical is to determine why there is such a wide range of responses among individuals.

There are many factors that can influence the glycemic index of a food," says Lichtenstein. "For example, a piece of white bread may have a high glycemic index but, if a person eats a slice of turkey and cheese with that bread, the effect of the multiple foods may result in a different glycemic index than if that person had eaten the white *bread alone. Since most food is consumed as combinations during meals and snacks, there is a need to assess the significance of using glycemic index values determined on individual foods for food mixtures. Similarly, it is important to know whether the food consumed prior to a meal or snack alters subsequent glycemic response*

-Tufts University, Health Sciences (2007, September 28). Glycemic Index Values Are Surprisingly Variable, Researchers Report. ScienceDaily. Retrieved December 22, 2008, from http://www.sciencedaily.com-/releases/2007/09/070926094725.htm

The other interesting thing that the study concluded was that combinations of foods can account for different insulin responses-- something that the Zone Diet also proposes. Dr. Sears suggests that fats and fibre are the two main elements in slowing down the absorption of carbohydrates in the blood stream. I recommend in the next section that you don't add any fats to your diet. You will get all that you need by accident, so whatever you do, don't eat something fatty because you ate a carbohydrate with a high insulin response. I did that for awhile, I honestly thought it would help me lose weight, but there are other factors at work, and the calorie density factor is one of them. Fats are high in calories and so are high insulin response carbohydrates. In this case, I was just swallowing the spider to catch the fly.

The answer is to not eat any of the high insulin response carbohydrates instead. I refer to these in general as the refined carbohydrates. I have a list below that shows the GI Index of many foods. The list is sorted from bad to good, using the same green, yellow and red coloring. The red items are foods that should simply be cut out or reduced in your diet to very small amounts. For example, I still eat a little bit of rice with my chicken some

black grey & white

days. It is a little amount, probably about 2 tablespoons (obviously rice is too sticky to try to measure 2 tablespoons when it is cooked, but it is about that amount). I still eat a little bread too.

Instructions for using **Table 5-4: Glycemic Index of Common Foods**:

avoid items in the black square (with a GI above 70)

If you eat them remember you are eating something very unhealthy and eat as little as you can. These are unhealthy foods.

eat items in the grey squares in moderation (with a GI between 50 and 70)

Eat these rarely and sparingly. They aren't good for you and they may spike your blood sugar levels. The only exception here is porridge, which you should consume 1/3 of a cup dry, for breakfast.

feel free to eat items in the white square (a GI below 50)

Note that meats will not increase your blood sugar, nor will vegetables. Use this chart in conjunction with the other charts in this chapter.

Table 5-4: Glycemic Index of Common Foods	
Name	Glycemic Index
White Rice	112
Potato (without skin)	111
Dates	103
Muffin	102
Pancakes	102
Cliff Bar Cookies and Cream and other protein bars	101
Sugar	100
Fruit Roll ups and similar snacks	99

Table 5-4: Glycemic Index of Common Foods

Name	Glycemic Index
Middle Eastern Flat Bread	97
Energy Drinks	95
Scones	93
Rice cracker	91
Sweet Potato	90
Popcorn	89
Honey	87
Pretzels, chips etc.	83
Cornflakes (and all other cereals)	80
Ice Cream	80
Watermelon	80
White Bread	77
Doughnuts	76
Jelly beans, etc	76
Pancake syrup	76
Crackers (varies average)	75
French Fries	75
Pancakes	75
Microwave popcorn	75
Cup Cake	73
Pop/soda	70
Spaghetti noodles cooked	70
Juices with added sugar	68
Jams with sugar	68
Pineapple, cantaloupe, raisin	65
Whole wheat bread	65
Raisins	64
Porridge (oatmeal)	62
Apricot	57
Bananas	53

MODERATE

Table 5-4: Glycemic Index of Common Foods	
Name	Glycemic Index
Cookies (varies average)	50
Skim milk	45
Oranges	44
Tomato soup	43
Pears	38
Apples	38
Boiled carrots	35
Grapefruit	25
Celery	15
Cauliflower	15
Broccoli	15
Tomatoes	15
Asparagus	15
Beef	0
Fish	0
Salami	0
Tuna	0

good.

Breakfast can be a dangerous place because of pancakes, syrup and high GI cereals. Other than oatmeal, there is one cereal you should eat. One cereal that is so full of good things, that I don't even think of it as a breakfast cereal any longer. It is All-Bran Buds. I sprinkle the buds on my yogurt, on my Oatmeal, on bananas and milk. It is a food additive to me, not a cereal. I will explain the benefits of this food in the section Fibre, coming up next.

There is a lot of talk about eating whole grains, as if eating whole grains will make you fitter. The point of whole grains really as that they are superior to eating refined grains with the bran removed. I don't agree with eating grains at all! I keep reading about the whole grain craze. Everyone should be eating whole grains, the USDA recommends three servings of whole grains every day. This is the new USDA recommendation by the way; it used to be way more grains and they didn't have to be whole.

I have a personal hate on for the governments dietary guidelines. In researching I have to be fair. Apparently it was way ahead of its time, and they did their best to recommend what people should be eating when people weren't getting enough nutrients, but for some reason, grains always ends up very high on the list. This is a list put out by the Department of Agriculture. I don't think I find this very surprising and I have to say that deep down I feel that the fox is in the henhouse here. I have spoken with many people and asked them, do you have to include grains in a balanced diet? Is there anything that we get from grains that we couldn't get from fruits and vegetables? So far, no one has been able to answer that one in the affirmative. As well, there are numerous other problems with the USDA's Recommended Daily Allowances but that isn't my issue here. So, instead of reading, eat whole grains, I want you to read, **IF** you eat grains, make damn sure they are whole grains. Otherwise grains are out of your diet for the most part. Whole grains contain fibre and that slows down the insulin response of the carbohydrate and that is better than no fibre at all, so that is why whole grains are better than more refined grains. But that is it. Foods made with grains are highly refined food products that pack a ton of energy into each bite For this reason you have to cut back on them drastically. I know you can't quite quit them, it probably isn't possible for most of us, nor truly necessary. How much you need to cut back is probably huge, but I will leave it to you to decide how you are going to handle them.

This is what I did recently, for example, when I was at breakfast this morning. I ordered bacon and eggs. It came with hash browns and toast. I know that eggs are a very well balanced food, so I didn't sweat that; I knew I could eat my scrambled eggs without worrying. I then had to look at the rest of my plate. The hash browns were bad. The toast was bad. This didn't mean I wasn't going to eat some of them. I couldn't not eat them. That said, I knew they were bad, so I only had a half a slice of toast with peanut butter and three or four small bites of hash browns. My kids always steal most of my bacon so I didn't get a whole ton of bacon either. You need to be able to recognize the bad foods and not eat them, or eat much less of them when you can.

For most of us, this process of eating better will be akin to a harm reduction strategy for drug addicts. We are probably not capable of going cold turkey on all bad foods. I know few people who can. I label those people fit people. They aren't like us (as I have been pointing out for the last 100 pages or so). For the rest of us, bad food is always going to be there, always singing its siren song to us. We just need to manage this so as to maximize our fitness. That we can do. We can be fit, look stunning in a bathing suit and manage our love affair with food. By having a bite of hash browns rather than an order. By having the backbone of our diet consist of healthy choices, we are much less likely to gain weight and much more ready to lose weight. As well, the less refined carbohydrates we eat, the easier it becomes to eat less. It really is a case of it becoming much easier to kick the habit when you aren't constantly battling cravings. Make sure to use the GI list in conjunction with the low food density list. A lot of websites have more information on both of these concepts; just remember to combine them both. To be healthy it has to be low in calorie density and low in glycemic index.

Fibre

For most of my life, and I mean almost all of it, I thought fibre was something that old people mixed with water so that they would be regular. I wasn't entirely sure what regular was, but I had a good idea it had to do with taking enough hmmm... how do you say it delicately...bowel movements? I didn't know if it firmed them up or softened them up, made them more common, or less common or what and why any of this mattered. Actually, now that I think about it, I still don't.

What I do know though, is that fibre is fundamentally important to your blood chemistry. Fibre slows the release of insulin in your blood. According to the Canadian Diabetes Association Fibre:

Combats constipation

•The most undisputed advantage of insoluble fibre is its ability to soften and expand stool volume, speeding up fecal transit and elimination.

Improves control

•Soluble fibre from legumes, barley, oats, some fruit and vegetables can help regulate blood sugar swings and by lowering serum cholesterol, protect against heart disease.

•Excess blood fats are possibly reduced by soluble fibres such as pectin, bean and oat gums, and the types in legumes (lentils, chickpeas, navy, pinto or kidney beans).

Heart health

•May improve by diets rich in fibre, through its cholesterol lowering effects.

Possible protection against cancer

•In the bowel, bacteria converts fibre into short chain fatty acids, which provide energy for the body and may help protect against cancer.

Fibre is one of those things that you don't hear anything bad about, and no large companies are trying to sell it, so you don't necessarily hear all of its benefits. It isn't like the battle between two giant fast food restaurants or colas, where there is no shortage of mind share that they are going after. It is one of those quiet yet often lauded tools for good health. Here has always been the playground of the fit people. We have always known fit people to eat high fibre foods. They have always had those sandwiches with the crazy breads that look crunchier than the crunchy peanut butter that you had between two big white slices of Wonder Bread.

A side note here about bread. Ironically, Wonder Wheat is one of the best whole wheat breads out there for you. The only mass produced one better in my opinion is Weight Watchers Whole Wheat. I find this story quite embarrassing but I will share it for its edifying value. When my wife first brought Weight Watchers Bread home, years ago. I was trying to figure out why it was better than regular bread. I read the label and I was amazed that each slice of bread had half the calories of regular bread. Half!! I was so impressed and I opened the loaf to pull out a piece of bread and the piece was literally HALF as thick as a regular piece of bread. This was no food engineering marvel!! This was no low fat, low calorie creation, this was just a sleight of hand. A trick!! I didn't eat that bread for years after discovering this. Until I started eating it. Then I discovered that regular bread felt too thick to me. I hadn't quite questioned why bread was as thick as it was (I think it had to do with the technology of bread loaf cutting machines at the time, but that is just a guess). I love bread, but I don't need more. There is a Wonder product out there called Texas Toast, quite aptly named, which is twice as thick as a regular slice of bread. It is incredible for french toast (something you should very rarely eat by the way, although if you are listening Wonder, I would love a whole grain Texas Toast, just for those occasions). Why is regular bread the 'proper' thickness for sandwiches and not Texas Toast? Who decided this anyways? As soon as I started using the thinner cut bread, I found out I liked it more. Then I realized this was the point of Weight Watchers Bread in the first place! I don't eat 2 slices of toast because I need more bread, I eat 2 slices of toast because my toaster has two holes in it. I don't eat 2 slices of bread with my sandwich because I want more bread, I eat 2 slices of bread with my sandwich because I want a handhold on both sides of my fixin's. My brother says he needs the second slice of bread for his sandwich as a cap, or a dramatic flourish to say his sandwich making is done and the eating can begin.

Since that time I have discovered that most of the new supermarkets have 'cut it yourself' bread-cutting machines. These things are awesome. I could spend a day cutting bread. If you are fast, and attach your loaf properly, you can vary the size of each slice from Texas Toast to just smaller than Weight Watchers (don't ask why you would do this. If you have to ask then you wouldn't understand, just use the bread machine to cut your bread as thin as possible). So, if you have a favorite local bread that is a whole grain bread, you can probably get it cut to Weight Watchers dimensions. The denser the bread the better for the bread slicing machine and be careful of bread too recently out of the over, it is tougher to cut thin. Seriously, by doing just this, you could cut your bread consumption in half and not even notice. As well, if you are going to whole grain, these two changes would be huge!

The number one source of fibre for you will be fruits and vegetables. You should get 26 to 35 grams of fibre a day, maybe more. The easiest way to get more fibre is eat more fruits and vegetables. The next easiest way is to eat All-Bran Buds. Each 1/3 cup of All-Bran Buds (yep, that is a pretty small amount of cereal) contains an amazing 12g of fibre. As well, these things will become very tasty to you. Obviously they aren't at first, but they will be. Again, this is just one of those "trust me" statements I keep making in this book. If you have followed along with me this far, just take my word on this one and go get a box. 12g of fibre!

Fibre Density

Below you can see the fibre density of selected foods. Fibre density is as important a concept as calorie density. Once again, you want good things from your food, but at what price? Certainly eating a bowl of Froot Loops to get 3 grams of fibre is a poor choice, so how do you choose what is a good source of fibre when products that don't contain much fibre can advertise that they are high in fibre? You have to calculate its fibre density. Any food that has a fibre density below 0.03 is not a good source of fibre. Don't eat it for its fibre. Everything between 0.03 and 0.05 is a moderate source of fibre, and everything above 0.05 is good source of fibre. Try to get your fibre from foods at the top of the list. Note, at the very top of the list, comes All Bran Buds with an FD of whopping 0.138.

Legend for **Table 5-5: Fibre Density of Common Foods**:

not a significant source of fibre (below .030)

light source of fibre (between .050 and .030)

a significant source of fibre (greater than .050)

Use this chart in conjunction with the other charts in this chapter.

Table 5-5: Fibre Density of Common Foods

Food Product	Fibre Density
Yogurt	0.000
All meats	0.000
White Rice	0.000
Wonder White Bread	0.001
Cucumber	0.004
Donut	0.005
Lay's Classic Potato Chips	0.007
Iceberg Lettuce	0.009
Peanut Butter	0.010
Brown Rice	0.016
Peanut	0.017
Bran Muffin	0.017
Almonds	0.019
Whole Wheat Macaroni	0.022
Wonder Wheat Bread	0.022
Newman's Own Natural Flavor Microwave Popcorn	0.023
Froot Loops	0.027
Cheerios	0.027
Newman's Own Light Microwave Popcorn	0.033
Raisin Bran	0.034
Campbell's Vegetable Beef Soup	0.038
Grapefruit	0.038
Onion	0.042
Orange	0.044
Apple	0.046
Pinto Beans	0.055

Table 5-5: Fibre Density of Common Foods	
Black Beans	0.055
Weight Watchers Wheat Bread	0.056
Strawberries	0.061
Refried Black Beans	0.064
Romaine Lettuce	0.067
Tomato	0.067
Lentil	0.068
Green Pepper	0.083
Broccoli	0.094
Celery	0.100
Cauliflower	0.100
All Bran Buds	0.138

So, remember fibre looks to be very good. I don't add any fibre powder to my diet. I don't know if it is a good idea or a bad one. I am leaning towards good, but I don't know if I would like the taste. If you start adding fibre to your recipes and find ones that taste good, feel free to send them to the website. If after review they appear to be healthy, I will post them for all to see.

Balance Carbs, Proteins and Fats

Your body needs Proteins, Carbohydrates and Fats to survive. There are several very famous diets that recommend that you reduce or eliminate any one of these elements from your diet in the short run to lose weight. What is arguably the most famous of these is the Atkins Diet. There is no doubt that these work in the short run, but they are simply diets. Actually, they are much worse than simply being diets. They are short term tricks that you play on your body. If there is anything you should have learned by now about your body, it is that you cannot trick it. It does not respond well to tricks. You convince it that there is no carbohydrates and you have to go through the difficult process of converting proteins to carbohydrates in your body and when carbohydrates return, your body will be much, much more efficient at converting those carbohydrates to energy in your body. This is the last thing that you want. So, take it as gospel that you need a balance of Carbohydrates, Proteins and Fats in your diet.

The question typically is how much of each. There is no definitive research on this subject and every expert is trying to make claims about his or her guesses. Of all of the works that I have read though, I have no reason to doubt that if the *Zone Diet* by Doctor Barry Sears is off in its calculations, it isn't by much. So if you want to know more about picking a diet based on exact amounts of macro-nutrients, pick up the *Zone Diet*. It is an excellent read and is full of remarkable scientific information to make his claims all the more interesting.

In any case, I am not here to give you complex calculations on how much of this or that to eat, because so far as I can tell, I have never seen a fit person do that. I have watched what fit people eat and they always eat a variety of foods that generally fall into the following categories: Low fat meats, plenty of fruits and vegetables, salads with a mix of vegetables and only a little non-creamy dressing, stir-frys, spicier ethnic dishes without cream sauces and fish.

So, here is what you should eat to look like a fit person. Eat low fat protein sources. These could include steaks, any fish, turkey or chicken or pork (ribs or salami, for example, should be eaten rarely). You want to typically eat about 4 oz (about 120 grams) of low fat meat with each meal. Yes, I know that is a paltry amount of meat. The reality is that the human body doesn't need a fraction of the energy you have been giving it. This is obvious, because you have been storing fat for awhile. So, you aren't going to get a hell of a lot of meat in your meal. How are you going to stay full. The answer is the low calorie density foods. Eat them with your meat source and you will feel full. Additionally, these items contain the carbohydrates that your body needs. Don't worry about eating enough fats. That just won't be a problem for you. Don't avoid heart healthy (unsaturated) fats, but don't try to add them into your diet. The reality is that you will add olive oil to your salads, and to your vegetables to cook them and you will get fats in your meats, so don't worry about adding fats.

The way I grew up doesn't help very much as well. I am fighting my whole life of eating now that I know that a balanced meal doesn't mean meat and potatoes, rice or pasta. For some reason every meal I have ever eaten has this balance. I am guessing everyone eats that way as well. You will have to get rid of the desire for this pairing. Once you give up potatoes and rice you really don't miss them, but kicking the habit at first feels like you are chopping off an arm. When I refer to a balanced meal in this book, I am referring to meat and vegetables. When I refer to vegetables in this book I am referring to those vegetables that don't include potatoes.

So a typical meal might be a half a grilled chicken breast on a vegetable salad (asparagus…), or 4 oz of grilled salmon with mixed seasonal vegetables, or a similar combination.

I have included a list of healthy food selections and recipes in the last chapter. These can be eaten at any time, for breakfast lunch or dinner (or for your fourth meal).

Additionally, Table 3-1 on page 30 has a list of healthy dining choices at fast food restaurants. Finally I am including here a list of entree choices at casual dining eateries.

TABLE 5-6: Healthy meal selections at Casual Dining Restaurants

Applebees

Chili Lime Chicken Salad

Apple Walnut Chicken Salad

Fajitas Steak or Chicken(get extra vegetables-tons of vegetables- and forgo the sour cream and cheese)

Garlic Herb Chicken (ideally hold the potatoes and get extra veggies)

Cajun Lime Tilapia (no rice extra veggies)

9 oz Sirloin with extra vegetables, no potatoes (Cut the steak in half and split the veggies into 2 parts. Take one half home with you)

Bourbon Street Steak (cut in half, get extra veggies no potatoes and take half home with you)

Chilis

Soup and Side Salad (soup is excellent for you as long as it isn't cream based. Get the house salad with a vinaigrette and this is an excellent meal with its own built in appetizer.

Quesidilla Explosion

Spicy Garlic and Lime Grilled Shrimp Salad

Classic Fajita, Fajita trio or steak and portabello fajita

Chicken Club Tacos or chicken tacos

TABLE 5-6: Healthy meal selections at Casual Dining Restaurants	
	Create your own combo with Grill Salmon, Margarita Chicken, Spicy Garlic and Lime Grilled Shrimp and Classic Sirloin (get extra veggies, and no potatoes. Split this meal into two halves and take one half home)
	Chili's Classic Sirloin (extra veggies, no potatoes or garlic bread, also hold the seasoned butter. Split this meal in two and take one half home with you)
	Margarita Grilled Chicken
	Guiltless Carne Asada Steak (split in two and take half home)
	Guiltless Chicken Platter (hold the rice extra veggies)
	Guiltless Grilled Salmon
	Guiltless Cedar Plank Tilapia
Olive Garden	
	Mixed Grill (extra veggies no potatoes, split in two and take half home)
	Venetian Apricot Chicken
	Grilled Chicken Spiedini

Water

A lot of experts recommend drinking 8 glasses of water a day. A lot of other experts recommend not drinking 8 glasses of water a day. You can find the argument for either side online. The point is without significant evidence one way or the other; we are going to go to the fit people and copy them. The fit people drink a lot of water. In fact, that is all that fit people drink. They don't drink much else. Sure, maybe a glass of wine with dinner, maybe a cup of coffee or tea in the morning and afternoon, but otherwise, it is all water all the time. For this reason, and for another much more important reason, we are going to drink a lot of water. The important reason is that water fills your stomach. This isn't to say that water fills you up, it doesn't really. Who hasn't been on some crazy diet where drinking water or juice is your main meal component. As anyone who has done that knows, that water does not make you feel full. What water can do is twofold. It can add to the food you are eating and make it feel much more filling. We know that we get enough calories in our food, probably too much and that is the battle that we are going to be fighting. So, when we can make less feel like more, we are winning. Therefore, have a glass of water with every meal. Every meal. Second, like the smoker who has quit his or her habit, you are going to get pangs of cravings constantly. You are going to find yourself in the kitchen all the time, with no reason for being there. Your body will just take you there and it is hoping you are going to grab some calorie dense food, even though you may not even be hungry. You are going to have an urge to do just that, even though you may not be hungry. Grab a glass of water. Sure, if you are actually hungry, grab a bunch of snacks on the below CD 1.00 list and eat those, but if you aren't feeling hungry grab a water instead and drink it. The craving will pass quickly and you will be fine. Start reducing your intake of diet pops if you switched to them from real pops earlier. I don't know why studies are showing that people who drink diet pop are as overweight as people who drink regular pop, but they are, so moving to water is a good move for now. Maybe science will explain this later. As well, when you find yourself in the kitchen looking for food, but not being hungry, ask yourself what you were doing right before heading into the kitchen. Keep track of this. If the same behavior keeps ending with you in the kitchen, it may be time to change that behavior. Your choice.

Action Plan

1.   Start reading the labels of foods that you are eating. Get nutritional information from all of the restaurants that you tend to eat at for the menu items you eat. Do this right away. Don't eat anything that you don't have the nutritional information on.

2.   Determine the calorie density of the foods you regularly eat. Figure out how they fit with the chart above. Try to eliminate or reduce the items in red and increase the items in green.

3.   Determine the GI of these same foods and do the same for them.

4.   Figure out how big 4 oz (100 grams) of meat is. Do this for beef, chicken, pork. Only eat that much of any portion. In restaurants eat one half a chicken breast and order an 8 oz steak and take half home. Ask for the vegetables with the meal, no fries, no mashed potatoes, etc. When you ask for the vegetables, remind them to hold the potatoes in the vegetable side dish as well, as there are always potatoes in those and ask them for more of the other vegetables.

5. Revise your recipes to match the lesson above. For example, if a recipe says it serves four, make sure it has 16 oz of meat in it and no more. Make up the rest in vegetables. Reduce the cream and butter in your recipes to get the calorie density down.

6. Add water to your routine.

Biggest Difference #5: Calorie Density of Foods

When you list off foods you love, nachos, burgers, fries, chicken wings, cheese sticks, etc are probably near the top of the list. When fit people list off the foods they love, salads, soups and stir fries are invariably at the top of theirs. This is simply a preference thing. I know what this is like because I have sat on both sides.

When I was younger I travelled around the South Pacific: Hawaii, Fiji, the Cook Islands, New Zealand, and Australia. The thing I noticed that was missing was vegetables. Stir fries and salads. They just didn't have them. There was so much greasy deep fried food. At first I was in heaven. Being a picky eater and getting tacos at Trader Joes in Raratonga was awesome. I had the greasiest, saltiest fish and chips and lasagna at one of the many take out places in Australia, and I can still remember those meals in Manley when I close my eyes. It was the best fish and chips I have ever had.

I was lucky enough to grow up with my mom feeding me some vegetables with every meal, usually a salad and peas or corn. The longer I travelled though, the more I missed the vegetables. I am sure it was just because I was traveling on a small budget that I never saw the healthier food choices, not going into high end restaurants and not cooking for myself, but in any case, I began to crave salads and vegetables.

On my birthday, one of the people I was traveling with, Heather, took me for dinner at the yacht club on the island we were staying on in Fiji. I was so excited when I saw they had a caesar salad on the menu. I ordered it and my mouth started watering. I was imagining the Hy's Encore Caesar salad that has always been my favorite. I have never been so disappointed in my life. The salad was a mixture of the toughest tropical greens (if you have ever walked on tropical grass you get an idea of how tough this salad was), with some lemon juice on top. I felt like the kid who ordered x-ray specs from the back of a comic.

So after 4 months of fast fried food and no vegetables I finally understood what it was like to crave food like a fit person. Think about this difference though, how much easier would it be to stay fit if you didn't crave the high calorie foods?

Deep fried foods really do taste disgusting if you aren't used to them. The breading is too thick and there is an overall greasy, heavy taste to them. But once you are used to them, the breading can never be too thick; after all, it is what soaks up the oil! Fit people just don't eat high calorie dense foods very often and because of that, they really can't stand them. By significantly reducing your deep fried and eating home made meals more often, you, too, could find your tastes changing to be more like those of a fit person.

Chapter 6
Organizing Yourself Like A fit Person

By failing to prepare, you are preparing to fail.
~Benjamin Franklin

Fit people are tremendously organized people. They are never caught without a pre-planned meal, nor without a full fridge. We rarely plan ahead, certainly not for food. They always plan ahead, especially for food. If you want to succeed at this, you are going to have to plan ahead.

That is one of the skills that they universally have. They organize themselves because they probably have had to their whole lives. They most likely participated in sports as kids, and had to get around to all sorts of sports destinations, prepared with equipment in hand. Whatever the reason, they are organized. Being so unorganized myself, this has always stood out to me, but what has also stood out to me is the fact that organization is essentially free.

Sure it isn't easy, and it is fighting against a lifetime of disorganization, but this isn't one of the traditional, frustrating battle grounds. This isn't exercise or diet, this is totally different and it has a massive impact on fitness. I want you to ask yourself that whenever you are having difficulty in one or more aspects of fitness, how much preparation did you put into it? How much planning? If you have failed at this point it is almost guaranteed to be a failure of planning. Plan to succeed this time!

A Little Background

I wish I had one story that could exemplify my complete lack of organization in life. I can't count the number of times I missed exercise sessions because I forgot my socks, or my shirt, or my shoes or my shorts. I have been 15 minutes late to swimming so many times because I have forgotten my goggles or my swim shorts, and I am lucky to live about 5 minutes from the pool where I swim.

Organization is more than a skill, it is a personality type. Unfortunately for us unfit people, it simply isn't our personality type.

A very big part of this book is learning the skills that fit people have and most of them are organizational. Last summer I competed in a sprint triathlon at Shawnigan Lake with my neighbor Jason. This involved an overnight stay and a ferry trip on top of all of the standard triathlon preparations. Jason's wife and kids came with us to cheer us on, and as it turns out make sure we were organized enough to compete.

Getting a ferry to Vancouver Island on the weekend in the summer is apparently much harder than driving down to the ferry and getting on. I knew this, but for some reason it didn't dawn on me until the day we were going to get on the ferry. Siobhan, Jason's wife, had already figured this out and called ahead and gotten us reservations. Hotels aren't any more available than ferries, but that didn't dawn on me either. There were half a dozen things that could have derailed my triathlon experience, and as such would have decreased my motivation to continue training. Not the least of which was checking to see if my bike was fine before we left. I had a flat tire on my bike before we left, something I could have and should have checked as part of a pre-race checklist, one of the many checklists I didn't have. The most important checklist you will need is a pre-workout checklist. There is one for many different activities at the end of this section, as well as on the internet.

Any number of areas where I failed to plan could have stopped me from competing on race day, but none of them did because someone who knew how to plan had already done all of that for us. You won't always have someone like that around. There are so many trite sayings about planning, such as 'failing to plan is planning to fail', but they are all true. As soon as you start planning to be fit, you will be amazed at what you can achieve.

Table 6-1: Weekly Training Checklist

Weekly Training Checklist

Task	Date	Date	Date	Date	Date	Date
Basic/Gym/:						
Running shoes						
Shorts						
Shirt						
Socks						
Shoes						
iPod						
Water Bottle						
Change for locker						
Toiletries						
Change of clothes						
Heart Rate Monitor						
Telemetry strap						
Membership card						
Towel						
Run (in addition to above):						
GPS/Timer						
Water belt						
Swimming:						
Goggles						
Swim suit						
Swim cap						
Change for locker						
Towel						
Trail Running:						
Camel Pack						
Shoes						
Cycling (in addition to basic)						
Bike Helmet						
Bike Shoes						
Bike test						

Law of fit people #6
Always plan ahead.

I know this law sounds a lot like law #3: Always Plan Your Food Needs In Advance, but this is different. Food planning is a daily activity that you need to get in the habit of. You will have 4 meals a day and you will probably have similar routines week after week.

Planning ahead in life is a lot more complicated. Life is complicated. People who find ways to be more organized are more likely to succeed at whatever they try. Planning has to extend to your training, but more importantly, it should extend to all of your life activities. You have a finite amount of time to get things done and the better you organize that time, the better your life will be.

Lesson #6: Get Organized

Organizing yourself to be fit involves two major elements, organizing yourself for your meals and organizing yourself for your workouts. You will find out how to do both in this section.

How to approach your meals

I have no idea how mealtime was in your house. For me there was a lot of eating in front of the TV, but almost always home cooked meals. Both my parents worked, so a lot of those meals had packages and cans to help, but they were still home cooked. We used to eat out about once a week, normally in a finer dining restaurant, rather than casual dining (there weren't many of them back then) or fast food. I racked my brain to remember what eating was like back then because I know it was healthy. I didn't start to gain weight until I was out of the house and in a different routine.

We had about 10 go-to meals (this is easy to say in retrospect, but we never had a meat loaf Thursday or anything, just that these meals were prepared a lot and enjoyed by all). The were:

- •Tacos (seasoning pack with shells and ground beef)
- •Spaghetti (seasoning pack and ground beef)
- •Salmon with rice and canned corn
- •Filet of Sole with rice and canned peas or artichoke
- •Roast Beef with potatoes and vegetables (typically canned)
- •Soup and Sandwiches
- •Shishkabobs
- •Pork Tenderloin with rice and vegetables (canned)

As well, there was always a salad before the meal. So that is about it. That is my go-to meal list of my youth. My mom was/is an excellent cook and my mouth waters when I think of the list. Why I am sharing all of this is because you need an easy to prepare go to list of meals. You need 10 items that you can prepare and do prepare regularly. **Whoever prepares meals in your family should have 10 healthy meals that you can eat.** Look through the recipes in this book and start selecting your 10. Think about the items you now prepare, and think about how you can make them healthy, then add them to the list. Every meal should have about 4 oz (112 grams) of meat (per serving) and a major, filling vegetable component (remember I don't define potatoes as vegetables, so don't ever think of them as such). Use the meat suggestions in the recipe section or convert any meal you currently eat to have a 4 oz. portion size per person. Select any of the vegetable dishes that I have in the back of this book (or on the web page) and mix and match them until you have your ten go-to meals.

Make sure you always have ingredients in the house for 2 or 3 of them and make sure that at least 2 or 3 of them can be prepared in 10 minutes or less. Make a list of these, keep updating it, and adding to it. It will give you some things to fall back on.

Print out or photocopy your recipes and keep them with your go-to meal list. Keep it in a handy place and use it.

Table 6-2: Go To Meal List

Go to Meal List
1.
2.
3.
4.
5.
6.
7.
8.
9.
10.

Weekly shopping list

If you are planning to succeed at being fit you need to have all of the tools of fitness at your fingertips. These are most often healthy foods in the house. We have already cleared out all of the unhealthy choices (haven't we?), so now we need to replace them with some healthy ones. There are some guides to this. Try to shop twice a week. One time to pick up nearly everything on your list (you can use the list below, but if you choose not to, make one of your own. You have to have a list), and one time to pick up some meats and vegetables. This is because most meats and some vegetables are only going to be good for about 4 days.

Make sure that your shopping list matches the list of 10 go-to recipes already discussed. These two items should mesh. For example, if most of your recipes have onions in them, make sure you always have onions in the house. As well, make sure that you have a couple of times like canned soups so that when all else fails you can always have a meal. Have a plan A, some fresh meals to cook; plan B, some leftovers to warm up from an earlier meal; and a plan C, some canned soups when all else fails.

Table 6-3: Weekly Shopping List

Produce	Seasonal Produce
Tomatoes	Corn on the cob
Lettuces	Berries
Cucumber	Grapes
Peppers-green	Avacado
Peppers-red	
Peppers-yellow	**Canned Vegetables**
Peppers-orange	Canned Peas
Asparagus	Canned Corn
Spinach	
Broccoli	**Deli**
Cauliflower	Sliced Turkey
Canned Peas	Sliced Ham
Canned Corn	other sliced meat:
Green Beans	
Celery	
Lemons	
Limes (optional)	**Meats**
Onions	Chicken breasts
Garlic	Steak
Carrots	Turkey
Apples	
Oranges	**Seafood**
Bananas	Salmon
Ginger	Halibut
	Trout
	Swordfish
	Shrimp

Frozen

	Vegetable Mixes
	Blueberries
	Misc. frutis

Canned Misc.

	Low fat refried black beans
	Soups

Dairy

	non-fat plain yogurt
	dessert yogurt
	Skim milk
	Goat Feta
	Egg Whites
	Eggs

Bakery

	Weight Watchers Whole Wheat Bread

Sundries

	Pickles
	All bran buds
	Oatmeal
	Pam
	Low-cal salad dressing
	Hot sauce
	Soy sauce
	Raisins

Others

you are ready to eat again. I find that at 4 o'clock, my mind is wandering a little at work. When I stop and grab a quick meal at my desk I am ready to go and I usually finish my day very well.

With regards to the snack before bed, there are arguments both ways on the eating before bed thing. Some people think that you shouldn't eat before bed because while you are sleeping you don't burn enough calories and you will store them. Others say that you should minimize the time between meals, and therefore eat right before bed. The thing that swings this argument for me is the fact that when you sleep you actually burn more calories than when you are sitting watching TV. Even if it is close (the difference in our BMR while watching TV and sleeping), this sounds pretty logical. It isn't like we are running a marathon after dinner every day. I find these arguments, that are based upon common sense statements, quite draining. You can spend hours at a dinner party arguing with other overweight people about things such as this. It must appear quite funny to the outsider. Here we are passionately arguing about a hair-splitting item that some 'celebrity trainer' has proposed, and yet we aren't even incorporating the things that we know work. If you find you are arguing a lot about issues that are fairly unproven, or unknown and you don't have a lot of personal evidence to back it up, think about other ways you could spend that energy getting fitter. If you come up with something, you are miles ahead! Think about this as well. These little changes that fitness experts claim will cause pounds to shed off your body, this little things that you are arguing with other people about. Are the people you are arguing with fit? Are the pounds shedding off them? I doubt it. Currently, and probably for the foreseeable future, there is no one trick to losing weight. It would be ridiculous to think there is.

In any case, it seems to me this eating before bed thing does not have a huge impact on fitness as there are still two sides to this story. If one side was distinctively better than the other I am sure we would have an idea about it by now. If you do find that you are eating food that you know is bad for you at a certain time though, change your routine. Eating potato chips before bed is bad (as is eating them ever). Switch to fruit, or change your routine so you aren't around chips in the evening.

Finally, the 4 meals a day plan has one exceedingly good quality. With 4 meals that are essentially nutritionally identical, you can switch them around any time. If you went out for lunch, cut it in half and took the rest back to the office for a later meal, you can eat that for your afternoon meal (I need to come up with a name for this meal by the way, I am leaning towards supper-although most people who use the phrase supper eat it as the last meal of the day, after dinner), your dinner, breakfast or lunch the next day. Whenever. Many times I will come home from work or a workout at 8 o'clock and have oatmeal and ham for dinner. More often than not I do this because I don't have any food in the house, or at least nothing prepared and I am hungry, but I have to say that oatmeal for dinner tastes great. This meal switching makes eating better so easy and that is why I really like it. I find my fridge is full of leftover meals that are great any time.

In many ways the 4 meal plan makes being organized easier, but you do have to commit to one more meal at a relatively inconvenient time. This is probably another meal away from home, so you may need to pack 2 small meals to work. If you are around the house during the day this additional meal becomes easier. In any case, organize your life so you can eat 4 meals a day. In the early stages of this organization, you should plan your meals, at least as many as you can.

So as much as I stressed making a date with fitness, you have to set some time aside to plan for good nutrition. Spend an hour, right now, thinking about how you can make your nutrition plans work for you. Write down what days you intend to eat what items. When are you cooking? When are you shopping? Use the chart on the next page to fill in this information. Include **every** meal and your intentions, cook a meal, eat soup, etc. Print up one of these sheets for each week and then make a goal to fill this in every Sunday (or whatever day you plan your meals and go shopping). Make sure you write it down. I probably don't need to keep reminding you of this by now, after all, you are a big person and responsible for yourself.... Okay, who am I kidding, I still have to remind myself. WRITE IT DOWN AND STICK WITH IT!!!

Table 6-4: Meal Planning Chart

	Breakfast	Lunch	Supper	Dinner
Saturday				
Sunday				
Monday				
Tuesday				
Wednesday				
Thursday				
Friday				

Rethink Appetizers

Appetizers have always been thought of as whetting your appetite. To whet means to excite or stimulate. That is the last thing we want our appetizers to do for us. We want them to dampen our appetite and this is what they can do. You know how they say that if you stop eating, in 5 minutes you will be full? It is true, it takes awhile for your mind to catch up with your body. To be full 5 minutes after eating, you should stop eating while you are still hungry. That is really hard though (bordering on impossible). One way to get around this is to eat a very calorie non-dense item before dinner, actually finish it 5 minutes before dinner starts. I highly recommend the apple. One nice big apple seven to ten minutes before a meal takes away that urgency that you may have with eating. So, have an appetizer; soups(non-cream based) and salads are excellent as well in reducing your overall appetite. Eat it 7 minutes before a meal. Think about it as replacing the high calorie items you usually eat. An apple is less calorie dense than french fries for example, but hot wings are not less calorie dense than salmon. Give the appetizer time to sink in, then eat your meal. By planning ahead with your meal, you can reduce your hunger.

Exercise organization

As much as you need to pre-plan your meals, you need to pre-plan your weekly workouts. Of course by now you have a plan so you know exactly when you are working out on each day of the week, but that isn't the end of your planning. You have to pre-plan your workout gear.

Are you going for a run? Is it outdoors or in the gym? Do you need to have a heart rate monitor? An iPod? Are you working out from home or from work? Are you going to work after your workout or coming home? The answers to these questions establish what exercise equipment you need.

Invariably for most workouts, you will need running shoes (cross-trainers are great all around shoes), a technical exerciseor cotton shirt, shorts or exercise pants of some sort, and proper socks. This is the minimum. If you are working out after work make sure you bring all of this with you. If you are working out before work, you will probably need a shower, so bring soap and shampoo and whatever toiletries you need to get ready. If you do this on a regular basis, go to the store and buy an extra set of all of these and put them together in a bag so you can grab them whenever you need them. As well, you will probably need a towel.

Having a travel bag for working out is great, but also keep a dirty laundry bag in the your workout bag for your sweaty clothes after your workout. You do not want to put them back in the bag. When you are working as hard as you should be for one hour, your clothes will be drenched in sweat and will get stinky in a closed exercise bag quickly. You are bound to forget them in there from time to time and that isn't pleasant.

The perfect exercise bag is one that you can pack with a week's worth of exercise gear and enough laundry bags for each workout. You need to have a spot for your iPod, your heart rate monitor, a stopwatch if you use one or your gps watch. You need to have a toiletries bag in there as well. There should be a mesh pocket for your shoes. Almost none of us have enough exercise clothes to fill a bag with all of our gear for the week. As well, I can't tell you how often I have been on my way to the gym and realized that I took my iPod out to charge it, or how often I have put on my GPS watch to go for a run and found the battery dead.

Seriously, not having your equipment ready to go for every workout will stop you cold. Take your time and make sure you have all of your equipment ready. Wash your clothes as soon as you get home and hang them to dry. They will be ready for your next workout. As long as your shoes are ready, your iPod is always charged and your clothes are clean, you should be able to stay organized for fitness.

Invest some money here to solve your biggest problems. If you never have enough clean clothes, buy some more. If you need shoes in your car and at home, buy 2 pairs. If you never have a charged iPod, buy a couple of iPod shuffles. Whatever it is that is holding you back, make sure you solve the problem. If you miss your exercise session twice in one month because of an equipment issue, invest some money in some more of that equipment.

Action Plan

1. You will have to shop at least once a week, and probably twice - plan on one major trip and 1 small one.

2. Use the shopping list shown earlier and make sure you have plenty of healthy food choices in your house and **NO** bad ones.

3. You should purchase some tupperware and plan to eat leftovers from dinner at lunch. If you cook some extra at dinner it doesn't take any more time and if you pre-pack it in a tupperware container, you will have lunch the next day.

4. Fill out your 10 go-to meals and keep updating this list. Keep it fresh while at the same time having your favorites around.
5. Plan your weekly meals in advance. Fill out a weekly meal form before you go shopping and keep to it.
6. Try eating an apple 7 minutes before your meal as often as you can.
7. Make sure you have time for meals and you have everything you need in place.
8. Make multiple copies of the per-workout checklist and customize it for yourself and how you work out (if you don't use a gps watch, cross it off the list).
9. Make a copy of your pre-event checklist and use it the week before your event, the day before, and the morning of.

This is the kind of organization and planning you will need to do on top of all of the other items in the this book. For example, make sure to give yourself time in the morning to have breakfast. Make sure you allow yourself this time because if you miss breakfast things will go badly for you. Every time I miss breakfast I screw up the day (although I did move enough breakfast items to the work fridge so I can usually do breakfast there).

To achieve this level of planning you will probably need to organize your family life well too.

Biggest Difference #6: Staying Up Late

Fit people go to bed early. We all have witnessed it at dinner parties. The first people to leave are always the healthy people. They drink and eat the least and leave early. Sure, they don't look like they are the happiest either, but they are always the fittest. So often, we stay to the bitter end, even planning a trip to the 24 hours drive through after. Do you not find it amazing that there are so many late night drive thrus?

This extends to late night television as well. Long after we should have gone to bed, long after everything we might have wanted to watch is over, we are still sitting there with the remote in our hand. Do you not find it equally amazing that after midnight there are so many channels dedicated to fitness infomercials and weight loss?

The market never misses opportunities to make money and that is why fast food restaurants are open late and late night TV is marketed to overweight people. They have noticed this habit of ours, this difference between fit people and the rest of the population.

Going to bed early has been shown in numerous studies to be associated with thinner, healthier people. There are many explanations for this, but it appears undeniably true given the sheer volume of research that has reached this conclusion.

Chapter 7
Take A Look At Yourself

Nothing can stop the man with the right mental attitude from achieving his goal; nothing on earth can help the man with the wrong mental attitude.
~Thomas Jefferson

Although you can read this book from cover to cover, this chapter is intended for after you have implemented all of the items in chapters through to 6. Until you have done your first event, and then read and begun to implement your improved eating plan, this chapter will not have a lot of value for you. This book is meant to be implemented in stages. This book should guide you along a couple of years of your progress. Yes, I could have just included a portion of this information in a book, and then added a sequel, but that would have felt disingenuous. After all, I wouldn't be giving you all of the tools that I have discovered to getting fit. That said, I will undoubtedly discover some more as time goes on, so I will keep adding those to the website until I have enough for another book ;-)

So, make sure that after you have some achievements and glory, that you come back and reread this chapter and the next two (in fact re-reading the whole book will be a great idea as you will have a different perspective on all of these issues). Do take your time learning these lessons by the way, and remember, trying to do too much too fast is the sign of being desperate, and you are no longer a desperate person. You are in this for the long haul. You know that success is assured, so don't run before you can walk.

You have made some serious choices and now have some control over your life. You may have gotten close to your final view of yourself. Now you can step on the scale (although you know the real measurement is how you look and feel, not what the scale tells you). Regardless of the real measurement though, metrics are important, so measure your weight. Use a body fat scale if you have one and write these things down.

A Little Background

Two years after my first realization, after my eye opening revelation, I was once again standing in the bathrrom. We had moved so it wasn't exactly the same bathroom, but it was mine. I was now 175 pounds and had been for quite awhile. I was working out once a week in the gym, running 10 km races twice a year and doing a sprint distance triathlon once a year. I was eating better, but I still enjoyed nights of drinking with my friends and most of my favorite foods, just a little less often. I was about 10 pounds overweight still, which shocked me, given how much more physically active I had been. Friends, trainers, everyone was telling me to just keep doing what I was doing and I would get down to my weight, but I realized this wasn't true. I had reached a plateau. For my level of exercise and eating, I had reached the weight that my eating and exercise balanced out to.

I hear people talk about plateaus and they consistently get them wrong. A plateau isn't a spot you are stuck on and as soon as you get over it, your weight will continue to come off. No, a plateau is the balance of exercise and eating and your current weight. At this level of exercising and eating you should weigh whatever you settle out to. This isn't a set point either, it is just your body.

Once I reached this point and realized just how much harder I had to work to go to the next level, I don't think I was really motivated to do it. I felt pretty good about myself and really didn't feel an overwhelming need to push myself further. That was when a very strong motivator came my way.

My trainer had sensed that I was pretty complacent with where I was. She challenged me to a bet to lose 12 pounds in 12 weeks. It wasn't a ridiculous bet and although she wanted me to achieve the goal, she wanted me to work hard too. If I won, she would take me out to dinner, if I lost, I had to pay for dinner and donate $500 to the charity of her choice. I did not have $500 to pay to a charity, certainly not after paying a personal trainer. I had to win that bet and I did.

I worked incredibly hard. In fact it was in this stage of work that I learned almost everything that I have written in chapter 9: How to Work Like A Fit Person. I became more diligent in what I ate. I drank less and I worked harder at the gym. I lost 16 pounds. I needed a small buffer just to be safe because weight can vary from day to day. I have never been fitter and it was great.

I had to make some significant changes to how I was living to get down to an athletically fit body, and you probably will have to as well, if that is something you choose, but for most of you I am guessing that being 10 to 15 pound overweight would be a glorious goal to shoot for. Once you get there, you can decide how fit you want to be.

A little note here about bets. Bets don't work twice. When someone sees your determination, they will probably steer clear of betting you again. Personally, I am very motivated by a challenge or by competition. Bets and competitions are a sure way to get me going. Here is a place where knowing your limitations and your abilities can really pay off. What is likely to get you working hard?

Law of fit people #7
Always focus on the long term, never the short term.

Looking on Twitter or talking amongst unfit people, I am constantly amazed at how unfit people only see fitness in the short term. They are always talking about diets and the more ridiculous and short term the diet the more excited they are. Fit people know that being fit means being fit for life, living a life with fit habits and activities.

This extends beyond fitness. Fit people know that success comes from looking down the road, not a week, or a month, but a year and more. When you change your lens to look at the long term, you can quickly realize why short term thinking won't solve many of our long term problems, if any. Stop thinking short term about fitness and you will be infinitely more likely to succeed.

Figure 7-1: Conventional Diets versus You Are Not A Fit Person

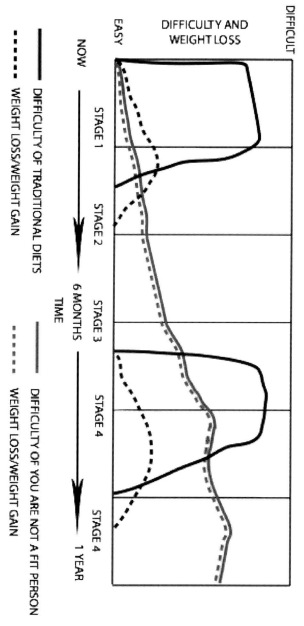

Lesson #7: Know the Difference Between Athletically Fit and Fit.

I think there has been a principle in my life that has simultaneously held me back and focused my abilities. I learned that I knew it (there are some things in life, you knew before you could put the words to them, for me, this was one) upon first seeing the film Dirty Rotten Scoundrels and hearing Lawrence Jamieson (Michael Caine) utter these words:

> *Freddy, as a younger man, I was a sculptor, a painter, and a musician. There was just one problem: I wasn't very good. As a matter of fact, I was dreadful. I finally came to the frustrating conclusion that I had taste and style, but not talent. I knew my limitations. We all have our limitations, Freddy. Fortunately, I discovered that taste and style were commodities that people desired. Freddy, what I am saying is: know your limitations. You are a moron.*

I spend a reasonable amount of time trying to understand my abilities. I have had to do this because I have racked up a considerable number of personal failures. I have had many successes, too, but the failures are harder to deal with. In my life I have taken on some pretty huge tasks. I have dreamed very big and believed that I could achieve those dreams. The problem was/is, I don't have a tremendous amount of follow through or stick-to-it-ness. This is a very bad combination. I remember in grade 5 for my science fair project I wanted to build a diesel engine.

I have no idea why, but I couldn't be swayed from my desires even after everyone pointed out to me how ridiculous it was. I ended up cobbling together a volcano at the last minute and putting in a home made smoke bomb (my brother showed me how to make them and they were unbelievably effective at making smoke) and getting a passing grade, but even later, by the time I took auto mechanics in high school, I couldn't put a lawnmower engine back together.

Originally I took this attitude to getting fit. I remember early on, I put up a poster of Carl Malone, a very fit basketball player to motivate me to become fit like him-if you have never heard of him, do an image search on google and you will get a laugh out of how high I set my sights. I probably thought I would get taller too. So I went after getting fit with the belief that I could be athletic. It didn't take me long to realize that I wasn't very good at achieving this. As a matter of fact, I was dreadful. For a long time I felt that I would never get fit because of this, but that simply wasn't true. I just needed to find what worked for me, and the only way I could do that was to know my limitations. You need to know yours if you want to succeed at difficult tasks and be happy doing it.

My limitations included the fact that I need to break my dreams down into bite sized tasks that will lead from one to another. I can keep moving ahead on small tasks if I am seeing verifiable results. Succeeding takes a while, and quite often it requires revisions to plans and goals, but if I keep at it, I do end up succeeding more often. More importantly though, I tend not to waste energy any longer on dreams that cannot be broken down into a trail of achievable tasks. Those are my limitations.

That said, don't let your knowledge of your limitations limit you. You can do more than you think. You are more powerful than you believe you are. That I guarantee, and that I will prove to you as we continue on this journey. Still, there is no healthy way to fit a square peg into a round hole. One of the keys to happiness in life is being able to tell whether you are pushing yourself to achieve something you should try to achieve or whether you are trying to do something that you cannot achieve. This is a lifelong pursuit of knowledge.

Carl Malone was an athletically fit basketball player. He was that fit because that was his life and he was paid millions of dollars to do so. Many athletes, models and movie stars are in this same position, but I am betting that there is one thing you didn't know. They rarely look as fit as you see them. During the off season, most athletes put on a few pounds and lose some muscle. Most models and actors go from fit to super fit right before a movie or shoot. Many models drop pounds of water weight the night before the shoot so their muscles and bones are more visible. This is captured in an image and in your mind forever more as a fit standard. Very few people are athletically fit all of the time.

To make matters worse, make up is used to accentuate muscles and photoshop is used to make people look leaner.

The point I am making is even if you are shooting for athletically fit, remember that there will be natural cycles involved. You do not want to, nor could you keep your body in such a distressed manner year in year out without risking it breaking down. You need to go through periods of rest.

Finally, getting athletically fit takes a lot of time. You may or may not have this time. Getting fit for living, though, takes a fair bit less time. You can make this time. So, if you shoot for getting athletically fit, don't quit if that doesn't appear possible. This isn't an all or nothing battle, but instead an incremental battle for your life.

Action Plan

When you reach a level of exercise and diet that you can maintain do the following:

1. Make a very clear list of all that you are eating and all that you are doing physically.
2. Compare this to your past charts.
3. Keep this handy and refer back if ever you feel you are going to slide. This is your fallback position.
4. When you are ready to push your fitness up to an athletic position, you are now ready to do so because you can safely stand at this level and come back here whenever you need to. You will never slip back to the unfit you.

This is the healthier you that you can live with. Never accept less than this. Now, if you want to go further, read on.

Biggest Difference #7: Love of Outdoors

Fit people love the out of doors. I see them all the time here in Vancouver. They talk about how great this city is with its winter sports: snowshoeing, cross country skiing and downhill skiing. Summer sports: hiking, rock climbing, cycling and ocean swimming. Of course, there is always the year round activities as well. They think of the value a city has based entirely on the things you can do that aren't indoors. I have always valued a city based upon the indoor activities it has.

I remember when I was young, some family friends of ours took us all hiking. It was rainy and cold and miserable. I hated it. I swore I would never hike again. Mind you, at that time in my life, watching TV was my favorite activity and remained so for most of my life. I didn't hike again until I was 37 years old. The first time I hiked as an adult, I ended up doing The Grind, a very famous climb up Grouse Mountain. It is grueling and an incredible challenge. From there I went to hike running. That is one of the ultimate work outs. Fit people have always understood that the out of doors is the greatest playground.

Us unfit people have a love of indoor activities. We love the TV and computer. Video games are a pass time for so many of us. When I was making video games, almost everyone in the industry was overweight, spent their time indoors, and rarely exercised. We just don't love the outdoors.

Chapter 8
Where To Go From Here

An hour of basketball feels like 15 minutes. An hour on a treadmill feels like a weekend in traffic school. ~David Walters

You have come a long ways. Congratulations, you have run your first 5k by now. You have created your fallback position, one that is based on the knowledge of healthy activities and healthy eating. You now know what exercise looks like and you aren't likely to get snowed by someone selling you a 3 minute fitness solution. So, where do you go from here?

Stick with your fitness goals, that is, your running, swimming, biking, triathlon, stair climbing, hiking or whatever your core fitness activity is. Follow your training plan, and get a new, more aggressive one each time you complete your goals. Do this and focus on your eating, continually getting a better grasp on what is healthy eating and what isn't, while getting into a more natural rhythm of eating this way. As I have always said (as long as Jeff isn't around to point out that it was he who always said this) that you lose weight through diet, not exercise. I do say though, that you keep the weight off through exercise.

In the past 3 years I have taken up swimming, running, biking, snowshoeing, hiking, cross country skiing and indoor climbing. I really enjoyed so many of these activities, at each one I met a bunch of great people and every one of those is an activity I can and do take my kids to, but at the end of the day most of these things aren't going to be part of my regular fitness routine.

The swimming though; I love the swimming and that has become the core element in my exercise. I think I will do it at least twice a week until I die. Because I like it so much, I am trying to constantly improve. I am in a masters swim class and I love the social aspects of that. We all hang out in the hot tub and chat for awhile after each class. I have gotten to know a bunch of the people from my swim class and I would consider several of them actual friends. This is how fitness ends up working for you.

This chapter contains some strategies on extending fitness in your life. When you reach this level, the fitness and the activities do become easier, but the key is to grab it and include it in your life. If you fail to do so, if you fail to embrace new activities and stick with them long enough to make them a habit, you will find yourself at your fall back position quite often.

A Little Background

Last year I signed up for an adult gymnastics class. Even to this day I am not sure what compelled me to do it. I think it was the memory of jumping from the mini-trampoline onto the mat in elementary school, along with all of the other apparatus that was set up in our gym. Something about gymnastics as a kid was fascinating and you really can't beat a sport that uses a trampoline. I don't know if I romanticized my childhood memories or if I really remembered it as a lot of fun, but for whatever reason the idea of jumping on and off stuff really appealed to me.

My kids were taking gymnastics and our community centre had installed a great new gymnastics centre just down the hall from where I do my masters swim class. I really like the idea of being able to see how hard it was to do some of the things my kids were doing. Turns out, what the kids were doing in gymnastics was hard, very hard.

I took 2 full sessions of adult gymnastics. For the first session I was the only guy. I liked that too. There were maybe 5 of us in the class and most of the girls had taken gymnastics as kids, loved it, never wanted to give it up, but did for some reason or another. Now they had a chance to take up where they left off. It was funny because everything they were good at, I wasn't and vice versa. I couldn't touch my toes even bending my knees and these women could still do the splits. I never really did cartwheels and round offs so that took me a long time, but the women were doing them like 12 year old girls. When it came to the vault and the bars though, I was so much stronger, which made up for the other difficulties.

In the second session though, some guys started signing up. Finally I could get a real comparison of how I was doing. The first thing that threw me was that immediately they all started calling me the 'fit guy'. These were ex-athletes for the most part and I was the fit guy! I was a little lower in weight than them, I had put on some noticeable muscles over the past few years and I look young for my age. Still this wasn't the only reason they thought of me as the fit guy. It turned out that I was faster, stronger and more coordinated than all of the people in the class (and this was after I just finished a grueling hour swim clinic). You can imagine my surprise. I have never been fitter than others. I have never been at the top of any physical endeavor, and now I was. After 3 years of running and training I had finally reached a level of fitness that not only did not hold me back, but actually vaulted me to an enviable top of the class position.

By getting fit, doors were opening all around me. From fun adult gymnastics to cross country skiing, I could do activities that I never would have tried before, and not only did I not fear that I would embarrass myself because I would be unable to fully participate, I actually found that I would be in the top half of any class I took. If you want to know how to get fitter, this is it. How many classes have you mentally turned down because you were scared you wouldn't be able to keep up? I have seen so many people who finally get the courage to try out for masters swimming quit because they aren't fit enough, and for each of those, how many never tried?

Once you are running 5k in under 30 minutes you are ready for so many activities that you would have been afraid of once before. These activities are vital to living a full life. I had no idea how many adult recreational sports and leagues there were. There are tons. If there isn't where you live, you can start one. When you are having fun and exercising, it is a positive reinforcement cycle that can't be beat. You exercise more because you want to be better, and you enjoy it more because you are getting better. Still this can only happen once you reach a threshold of fitness.

What is holding you back from signing up for clinics to run further, classes to learn new skills, or groups who share activities? You are so close to the top of the hill in fitness here, reach out and grab the flag.

By the way, the adult gymnastics class was fun, but after 2 sessions (8 months) I was done. The first thing that I remembered after starting the class is why I never enjoyed gymnastics as a kid. Sure, the equipment looks fun, but you have to go back and do the same thing over and over and over again until you get it perfect. I don't care about perfection and I never did. I am happy I can just somewhat do it. I grew very bored in the gymnastics world. As well, my injury prevention coach had advised me repeatedly that I should not be doing adult gymnastics. He would do this with a look of shock on his face, shock that I had ever signed up for something so dangerous.

It was dangerous too. We did all sorts of crazy stuff, and to my mind, the craziest was front handsprings off of the vault at full speed. It just didn't dawn on me how crazy that was, until after I failed to roll out of a simple handstand and landed on my neck. I shook it off and pretended that it didn't hurt, but in my head I was screaming in pain and wondering if the pain would ever stop. Of course I didn't want to look like the idiot I was, so I got through the end of the session, and then iced my neck and shoulders. It took quite a few weeks for the neck and shoulder pain to go away and I realized that adult gymnastics was potentially interfering with my goals, the goals of being a fit person. As well, I realized that I wasn't as young as I felt. If I ever think about signing up for adult gymnastics again, I just think of how foolish I looked slumped over, head first on my shoulders with my head at a 90 degree angle and my legs splayed above. That is not the road to fitness for me.

If adult gymnastics is a goal of yours though, and it is an excellent goal, then go for it, be careful, and take every precaution you can to be safe. Attempting to do the iron cross on the rings was incredibly fun and challenging and that challenge makes training for rings an unbelievable activity.

It turned out not to be my goal, but still, it was great to know that I could do adult gymnastics and be stronger than everyone there because I had followed the plan that I have outlined above. There wasn't anything holding me back physically from a great performance.

Law of fit people #8
Be good at what you enjoy and enjoy what you are good at.

I have seen this time and time again. Fit people are the people who were excellent at the sports and activities they did as children and this is why they stuck with them and became fit. Who wouldn't do what they are good at, and who doesn't enjoy doing what they are good at? It is so simple, yet we miss the importance of this time and time again.

Having children, I have had the opportunity to see them participating in active field trips with their school; most recently a series of 3 cross country ski trips. Cross country skiing isn't an easy activity and it takes strength and coordination. At ages 9 and 10 the spectrum of abilities is amazing. The kids were broken down into 10 groups of about 10 kids each and in each group you tended to have about 6 kids who were at about the same level, 2 that struggled a little and 2 that struggled a lot. Each week you knew that the 2 that struggled a lot would not be coming back the following week. Strangely there would be 2 more that would struggle the next week. I could tell you before the session started who these kids were likely to be and I will predict now that each and every one of them will turn away from sports and activities in the next year or two--if they haven't already--and they will take to computers and TV instead. I know because I was one of these people.

We have governments asking why we are obese and the answers are all right here. Make fitness fun for everyone, get rid of the stereotypical 'Mr. Woodcock' fit person gym teachers, and spend some money creating more levels of training that allow everyone to be at the top of their class for a while. Those are ideas for our children, though; for us that ship has sailed.

The problem we have is that if you don't enjoy it, you won't do it, so although you may not be good at it, or traditionally not have been good at it, now you have to find ways to enjoy fitness regardless. Some things you can do is make sure you are at the top end of your group in terms of fitness by either choosing a weaker group to be in or getting yourself fitter. You can participate in individual sports until you get fit enough to join groups, or you can stop caring what other people think and just have fun. If you decide to follow this latter plan, which I am a huge fan of, make sure that you don't get in the way of the people who are at the generally accepted level of the group. Just pay a little more attention to being polite and finding ways to not slow everyone down, and remember to have fun!

Lesson #8: Clinics, Gyms and Classes

Extending your out of gym routine

Once you have confidently completed an event, then you may be ready for a clinic. Look around for clinics that are about your level and trying to achieve a goal that you are working on. If there is a clinic around that you can sign up for to get ready for your next event, do so! You can't beat a clinic.

At this point in your fitness a gym membership might make sense. If the weather is seasonal where you are, using gym fitness equipment can keep you active longer and resistance training is an excellent way to push your fitness forward.

When you are signing up for a gym, think about signing up for a regular class there too. The gym isn't the only place that offers classes, though, so look around.

Clinics

What are clinics and how do you find them? Clinics are group training programs that work towards some shared goal. There are walking clinics, running clinics, biking clinics, swimming clinics and triathlon clinics. These are for many different distances. Clinics are led by experts and enthusiasts who enjoy sharing and who have a wealth of tips and advice. As well, you will participate with people who share your goal. Now that you have done some work on your own, you will probably be in the middle of the group of people who participate in a clinic. Some will be healthier, some will be less healthy. This will feel great. You won't worry about your fitness level holding you back any longer, and you will be part of the fitness group. You will bond with some of the people in your clinic and you will want to beat others. The desire to beat others will probably drive you as much as anything.

These clinics are the number one way to move ahead in your fitness. If there are clinics in your area, look into them and sign up for one that you definitely can attend. Clinics in Canada are typically put on by running shoe stores, swim gear stores or bike stores. The Running Room puts on clinics all across Canada and on top of the fantastic clinics, they also have some neat features, such as pace bunnies. These are volunteers who run in the race your clinic is getting ready for, and they run at a set pace, which is written on pink ears that stick up. That way you can visually keep a pace that you need to keep to stay on track. It is brilliant, and although I don't know if they were the first to do this, I would hope that other clinics, clubs and even races could follow suit. My local shoe store is North Shore Athletics. They put on some fantastic clinics and a friend of mine signed up for the triathlon clinic last year. She was quite overweight and had very little fitness experience. She was recently divorced as well. She not only competed in a sprint triathlon 3 months after starting; with her clinic group, she went on to compete in an olympic distance triathlon 3 months after that. To say that the fat just melted off of her would be such an understatement. I have witnessed this. Clinics are awesome. The people she met, the people she got to know, the support and the desire to beat others in her group drove her on to mind-numbing successes. I can't wait to see what the next year will bring for her.

In the US running clinics are typically put on by running clubs which can be searched for online.

In Europe, it looks like trainers and running clubs alike offer clinics.

If you don't find a club in your area there, search the internet. If you still can't find a clinic, talk to your local college or high-school. They may have a track club and members of the club might be willing to put on a clinic. If all else fails, start your own. Post some fliers with your phone number and start a running club. Use one of the running training plans that I have supplied and follow it as a group. Although I don't recommend training with someone at the beginning of your fitness plan, now I think you want to become more involved with people who share your goals. Early on you can hitch your wagon to a falling star and end up failing because of this. Now you have shown yourself what you are willing and able to do, and that momentum will probably keep you going even if you should start training with a quitter. Your determination will keep you going regardless. That said, if you select a training partner who drops out, you are certainly more likely to quit, so find a clinic, join a clinic, start a clinic. After all, you will have many people to work out with and that will definitely keep you going.

The Gym

We are going to take some of our training indoors. The gym is a great place to work on our muscles. Why am I saying this? Didn't I earlier say that the gym was a hard place to be? Yes I did. That was then though. Now, you have a goal. Now you have an 'out of gym' program. You are going to **use the gym to strengthen that program**. You are going to add resistance training to your program and hopefully, if all goes well, develop a home base (by home base I mean a location that is outside of the home but feels like your home away from home with people you enjoying seeing on a regular occasion), an indoor location with access to cardio equipment and training sessions. Your 'out of gym' program is going to be your go to program, so the gym will just be in addition. This is a great opportunity to develop some muscles for show and as your fat decreases, your muscles will begin to show. As well, this gives you a chance to broaden your fitness experience, again giving you some more potential experiences that may stick. Here it isn't a question of cardio or resistance training. It isn't a question because the answer is both. Both to improve your fitness so you can compete at a higher level at your aligned goal.

Finding a Gym

There are a number of different types of gyms that you can join. Some are better than others, but at the end of the day you are going to have to decide for yourself which is the one for you. Remember that variability over individual gyms will be greater than variability between chains, which is to say, there may be good chains with some bad gyms that happen to be near you, and there may be some bad chains with great gyms near you, so make sure you pick the gym not the chain, no matter what you hear about chains overall on the internet.

There are 4 types of gyms in general. The College, YMCA or Community Centre gym is the easiest to access and has the lowest pressure sales team trying to get you to sign up. These typically allow you to pay a drop in fee rather than sign up long term, which is nice. If you can afford a boutique gym, that is your best bet. Typically you pay for personal training sessions and have access to the equipment whenever you want. These gyms truly become a home away from home. The chain gym is very common and typically offers all of the services and equipment you could want. Finally, the boxing/fitness gyms are similar to the boutique gyms, but they typically have one or more fitness angles that are unique to them, such as MMA or Boxing. A list with examples is below:

College Gyms, YMCA's and Community Centers
> Universities
> Municipal gyms and pools
> Boys and Girls Clubs

Boutique/Personal Training Gyms
> Innovative Fitness

National Chains
> 24 Hour Fitness
> Golds Gym
> Bally Total Fitness

Boxing/Fitness Gyms
> Lava Sport and Fitness
> Sugar Rays Boxing Gym
> Griffin Gym
> Crossfit

You need to pick a gym that you can afford. Most gyms have some start up costs that they bundle up into an annual contract. Most of the prices of gyms can be found online along with what they offer. Check out the contract time and conditions before signing anything. With the bigger gyms they will all require you sign a contract that includes a time period that you will be a member for. For these gyms, from what I can tell, you are looking at about $40 a month, with a one year commitment. If that is too much money for you, then seriously think about the YMCA, college gyms or Community Centre in your area. These are normally great facilities and many offer all of the same things as the chains. If you can't afford these solutions, then realistically, you are going to have to focus on upping your out of gym training.

Almost every gym will allow you to try it out, with the larger chains giving you a week to explore it at least. Do this. Never join a gym without trying it out first. There are a million factors as to whether a gym will work for you. What is the atmosphere like? Is it intimidating? Maybe a community centre would be a better fit. Are the people fit enough? It is nice to have some eye candy around when you are working out, and the hope of meeting some of these people will probably bring you back more often than anything else. Are the people like you? Finding people in the classes that share your values is really important. Feeling like an outsider at your gym will probably stop you from going. Also, you don't want to be the least fit person there either. On top of how the people look at the facilities, are the facilities clean? How many machines are out of service? This happens at the best of clubs, but what percentage of machines are down? If it is a lot, you might want to keep looking. What other things do they have? A swimming pool is nice, but not a necessity if you can swim somewhere else. How about racquet sports? Again nice. How are the trainers and the people behind the desk when you get there? They are likely to be fit people, so don't expect to want to be their best friends, but are they knowledgeable and helpful, or are they trying to sell you the latest supplements and clothes? Can you at any time ask for assistance in the proper form for a new exercise. This is critical. Most weight training exercises, when done wrong, will result in injury, but some will guarantee injury with even the slightest errors in form (standing rows, dead-lifts and power squats come to mind). If you are ever doing an exercise for the first time, get a trainer to help you. Also, check in from time to time with a trainer to confirm you are still doing it right; some errors in your form may creep in as you work out.

Multiple locations are great if there are locations near your home and your work, as well as other places you may spend a lot of time. That said, if your house is near your work and both are near your gym, you may not need multiple locations. I can't stress enough how important it is to pick a gym that is nearby your daily life. **The location of the gym is in my experience the number one determinant of whether you will use it.**

It is very important that the gym that interests you has plenty of group exercise sessions or classes. I am going to strongly recommend that you sign up for group sessions and you can see that below under classes.

Your gym should have several treadmills and ideally some treadmills located in the gym with 1 hr time blocks. That way you can run about 10k without any reason to have to get off the treadmill. Check out the gym several times during a week, at likely times for you to work out, and see that they have enough cardio equipment for you. Smaller more boutique gyms need a lot less equipment than the larger gyms to ensure that you have access to equipment. Therefore the actual number of machines isn't as important as looking at the machines during different times, and judging how busy they are. Obviously 3 treadmills for 60 people is much much better than 30 treadmills for 6000. Also, don't try to judge any gym in the first two weeks of January. I have never been able to get a parking spot within a mile of my gym in the first two weeks of January, let alone a treadmill. This is the super peak period, the 100 year storm of gyms, if you will. This is the New Years Resolution crowd.

Here are some additional tips that I got from Melissa Tennen, HealthAtoZ   writer (http://www.healthatoz.com/healthatoz/Atoz/common/standard /transform.jsp?requestURI=/healthatoz/Atoz/hl/fit/star/alert090 22004.jsp)

I never would have thought of this as I am not a fit person, and I tend not to plan perfectly (I tend to just jump in), but make a list of all of the gyms in your area. I would go further to recommend you create a matrix on a sheet of paper (a table showing the gyms in a column with the features that interest you in a row at the top). That way you can compare features directly in making your decision. All that said, you will probably just find one you like, that works, and go with it, but I can't ignore this great fit person advice and not pass it on to you....

Ideally, you want to go to a facility with certified trainers. That said, not all regions have certifications and not all certifications are the same. You can ask your gym if they have certified trainers and then ask them what their certification is. You can check the validity of this certification online. Because there is no law protecting the use of title or practice, anyone can call themselves a personal trainer and anyone can act as a personal trainer, so it is very important to find out what training and background they have and what qualifications. Certification is your best bet here, but talk to the gym.

Finally, contact your employer or your health plan provider. As Melissa Tennen points outs, your company may have a co-pay option at some gyms. If someone is paying for part of the gym, that is a no brainer.

Resistance Traning

There isn't enough room in this book for me to share all of the required information regarding resistance training techniques that you are going to need for your life in the gym. This is because changing your program when you are doing resistance training is very important. I will recommend the best books on resistance training in the appendix. I highly recommend that you periodically get a personal training session from time to time to learn new techniques and check the techniques you are already doing (see personal trainer below). If you can't afford them, ask for them as birthday presents, etc. There are always gift certificates that all gyms have and it will give your friends an opportunity to take a part in your fitness.

Classes

Classes are key. Classes are awesome. They are typically 1 hour in length (this is a good length for a workout). They have the potential for a social aspect, meeting people, and getting to know others who are doing the same workouts you are. There are a bunch of great classes at all of the gyms. You need to get your heart rate up into your cardio zone for about 40 minutes, so you will want to pick your classes based on that (see Training in your Target Heart Rate Zone for more information on your cardio zone). Find a class that is good for your schedule and that you enjoy. Spinning classes are great. Any of the body sculpting, weight bearing cardio, boxerfit classes are excellent. Make sure that the classes that you will use are included with your membership. As well, make sure that you make an appointment with your class. Seriously do not miss it. Find a class that you like. Here you are adding your out of gym workouts with one or two sessions in classes, you will see remarkable improvements in your body composition and these classes will very often improve your out of gym training and your fitness base.

I think that if you commit to a class you will find that it is the thing that you keep doing when all else fails. As soon as you are ready, take a regular class and stick with it for awhile. If you don't like it, try another. Don't give up; you will find the class and the activity that is right for you.

Home Training

I know a lot of people who prefer to train at home. They buy an exercise bike or a treadmill and go at it at home. I have no problem with this if you have kids and plan to run after they are asleep or some other strong commitments, but if your intention is to do your training at home because you don't like gyms or feel out of place training around other people, then you are just making this harder than it needs to be. Really, the social aspects, the classes, the meeting people and the feeling of actually getting out and doing something are all fundamental to your success. Again, this isn't easy. This is a life long battle. You need every possible variable in your favour.

So, if you are using a home training device on top of your 'out of gym' training and your classes, etc, then bravo. There are quite a few options here for you to choose from. Theses include:

stationary bike

Low impact and quiet. This is a great home machine, especially if you have one that has programs for uphill and downhill.

treadmill

A treadmill is always a winner. It is louder than a bike by a ways; it also takes up more room. That said, it allows you to run year round and running is the best exercise. Also treadmill running is softer on your knees than pavement running.

Elliptical

The Elliptical trainer is a fantastic, low impact, all over body exercise because of the additional hand holds. I have never really enjoyed working out with them as I find the motion quite odd and I have a hard time getting motivated while using them. I have no frame of reference on how hard I should be working, how hard is good. That said, my neighbor Jason recommended that I wear my heart rate monitor next time I use it and pay attention to how hard I need to work to stay in my training zone. It is a great idea and I think that the elliptical may become the backbone of my gym training. Careful when purchasing one though, some elipticals are actual circulars and that motion is no good on your knees.

Stairmaster

The stairmaster is the gold standard of cardio building machines. It can be quite grueling and boring as well. Still, if you wanted to get your cardio up to its strongest in the shortest time, the stairmaster is the machine for you. I loved watching my improvement on a stairmaster. It was a lot of fun. That said, there was nothing else fun about it. The stairmaster is a machine with pedals that go up and down. There is an awesome stairmaster, called a stepmill that looks like a 3 stair treadmill. These are probably a little expensive for a home gym, but they are even harder than the stairmaster. I prefer them, but they are much, much harder to run on as well. I keep having to look down, and you don't want to look down while exercising.

Spinner

The spinner is a stationary bike with a large fly wheel in place of the front tire. This fly wheel mimics the real feel of cycling remarkably well. Remarkably. This is an excellent training device, especially for those serious about bike training. There are some videos out there that you can buy and play that will help give you a program like a spinning class in the privacy of your own house. One warning with these; the pedals are directly connected to the fly wheel, so when you stop pedaling the pedals don't just stop like a regular bike. I have almost looked like the biggest idiot in the gym on many occasions by forgetting this fact.

Bike Trainer

The bike trainer is a fly wheel device that attaches to the back wheel of your bike. This is for the triathlete or serious cyclist only. This gives you the most realistic indoor training option possible. You can do the training on the same bike that you are going to be competing on, and you can buy many videos with programs you can play while training. This is a great option for an in home device, because it can keep you active training for events that you are going to be doing later in the year and you can do it directly in your house. The training sessions can get a little boring though. That is the case for any indoor training, to be honest. This will become more and more of a problem for you the more you actually compete and train outdoors. The variety and visceral experience of training and competing outdoors will be part of what keeps you exercising throughout your life. Training indoors is hard to keep doing, without a very strong goal. Still, coming into a year with a good cycling base will massively improve your triathlon times, so sometimes you must suffer to get the most out of yourself.

Swiss Ball

This is the only non-exercise machine I am going to mention here. The swiss ball is excellent. It is a great item that can be used to improve your posture, and equally importantly, to work on your core muscles. For this reason you can get and use a swiss ball in your daily core muscle exercises. Otherwise, all of the other fitness items that you may think of are just tools. Do you need them in your tool kit? Probably not. Do they work? Maybe, but will you use them enough to justify buying them? That is doubtful. Doubtful in the extreme. So I don't recommend the investment. A skipping rope is an excellent training device. I have 2. I don't use them. I wish I did. The problem is that they are so damn exhausting. You really can't skip for very long. It is brutal. So you don't get it out as often as you would like, and after awhile you don't even know where you keep it. If you have always wanted to skip rope and you think you will use it and you have a spot to use it, then by all means buy it. If you use it, that is awesome. If you don't you are only out $5 to $19. In fact, many great exercise devices are pretty cheap, so as long as you have your core, 'out of gym' training and a few gym sessions a week, you won't lose focus or drive by getting exercise equipment and not using it. You can find instructions on how to use this equipment on the net, as well as reviews and information about what works and what doesn't. Just remember that each of these items is a tool in a tool kit. Many are highly specialized. None of them will build you a fitter body on their own. Like any person who has a tool kit and loves getting tools, many will never get used, but that doesn't mean we love our tools any less.

Action Plan

1. Extend your fitness activities to include at least one new competitive activity and one new recreational activity every year.
2. Include your family.
3. When you find competitive activities you like, hire a trainer with some knowledge of that activity, go to the gym with the trainer, and learn to be more competitive.
4. Look around, find, and sign up for clinics and classes.

Biggest Difference #8: Physical Activity

For whatever reason as we grew from childhood we have moved away from physical activity probably because we were getting progressively worse by comparison with others.   At some point this mattered and we stopped participating in the activity. I can remember when I stopped, and I don't know if it was just that I sucked at sports or that I didn't really enjoy them, but there is a great likelihood those went hand in hand.   I never received accolades and compliments for what I did, so I went off to do things I enjoyed more.

Fit people did receive those accolades and compliments. They enjoyed the activities and stuck with them.   They stayed fit, participated in tons of different activities, and physically developed to be better at all sports. Fit people can pick up just about any sport and excel at it. They never lose this ability, although it certainly gets rusty. They are always in the top half of the people doing any fitness activity and they are never afraid to compete on this battlefield. We are.

Fit people put a priority on physical activity. When given a shortage of time, exercise is always at the top of the list. This includes the fact that fit people go to bed much earlier on average than un-fit people. This allows them to get up early and get in some exercise. If you can exercise first thing in the morning, then you are very likely to succeed at fitness. I never have been able to do this. I will always choose to stay up a little longer, working or watching TV rather than going to bed to get up early. If you were to write down your top 10 priorities on a sheet of paper, from most important to least important, and compare this to a fit person, the most glaring difference would be exercise. We all place a high priority on family and work, but after that, what is the next item on your list? For fit people it is exercise.

Once you open the door to fitness, you are no longer in the bottom half of any class that you enter, unless you reach for the best classes, and well done if you do!! You really will be well on your way to being a fit person if you stick with an activity that you don't excel at, because you enjoy doing it regardless. I know that is how I approach swimming. I have been the worst swimmer in my masters swim class for 2 years (don't ask me how I have achieved this, I am not sure myself). I really am not improving compared to the people I swim with, and no one worse than me is joining. The interesting fact, though, is that compared to people who aren't in my class, I am getting so much better!

By the way, most unfit people play golf. We think we enjoy it because we are competing against ourselves, but that really isn't the main reason. When you play golf, most people don't hit below 100. One hundred isn't very good and most people can do this with a little practice. When we are golfing, we are typically with a foursome and it is easy to find 4 people who are relatively competitive. In golf we have just isolated ourselves into a small matched group to compete against. If every sport were this way, with the bulk of the players being relatively average, and the competitive groups being extremely small, we would be infinitely more fit. Everyone loves to play games, have fun and maybe even compete with people who are at the same level or slightly lower.

Chapter 9
How To Work Like A Fit Person

Effort is only effort when it begins to hurt. ~José Ortega y Gassett

So often I would go into the gym and not work that hard. Sure I thought I was working hard, but in one way or another I was fighting against the experience, against the idea of doing more. I listened to my body when it said I couldn't do another rep or set. I spent an extra 10 minutes at my desk or home before going to the gym, because I just didn't want to go. I never rushed, I never pushed harder than I had to.

This is not how fit people approach fitness. Every day I see people saying that they don't understand why they are overweight. This chapter is the answer. The fact is, fit people embrace so much that we avoid. When you actually see how hard fit people work out, you no longer ask why am I not fit. You will know why. You will know what it takes to have an athletic physique. Amongst fit people this is called 'getting it'. When you 'get it' you get it. You are clear on what kind of work it takes to develop six pack abs. You don't need to ask anymore. You know how much help in terms of support and training you need to get the most out of yourself.

This chapter teaches you how to work out harder with instructions on creating an objective method for measuring how hard you are actually working. You will learn how to fuel yourself for a workout and how important this is to getting the most out of yourself. I will share with you the value in using a personal trainer to get even more out of your workout, and finally, you will find a myriad of additional tips on how to work out like a fit person.

A Little Background

I can clearly remember the day that I saw Shauna running on the treadmill at Innovative Fitness. Shauna was a trainer there and she is a phenomenal distance runner. Innovative Fitness hired exceptional athletes and people from many different backgrounds, and really the main thing they had in common was their drive for self improvement. At Innovative Fitness you did your profiling once every three months to measure your progress, but the coolest part was that the trainers did this profiling as well. There would be a 1.5 mile run, push ups, sit ups, chin ups, burpees, timed plank and a number of other painful routines that were measured and compared with past performances. You can see just how much more effective this would be to keep track of than just weight loss.

So on this day I noticed Shauna running on the treadmill. She was flying along, but people running on a treadmill never look as fast as you think they would. In any case, I was just starting my workout, I was warming up and I noticed how hard Shauna was pushing herself. She worked right through the pain (this isn't joint pain or injury, but that loud voice inside your head saying. 'Stop-- this hurts....' Yes the one you used to listen to). Her face turned red and she got a very far away look in her eyes and she pushed on. At this point everyone had begun to cheer her on and push her to run harder and 'finish strong', including me.

I was in awe. I have never been so near someone giving their all. I had known of people who did. I know my trainer had won some 10k races, races I ran with her. I am sure she pushed herself this hard, but by the time she was coming around to the finish I was about 5 kms behind (I am not exaggerating).

I learned that day just how fit people workout. Just how hard they are able to push themselves, and I was able to use that knowledge to push myself much further than I ever thought I could.

Law of fit people #9
Never listen to your mind when it says you are hurting or can't go on, it is wrong, you have much much more to give.

This is a lesson that quite simply cannot be learned easily, but it is a lesson deep down within each of us. I am no longer surprised at how much more I can do when I am called on to do so.

Last year Meyrick and I were filming an exercise segment for a reality TV show we were on. Meyrick had grabbed some weights and was doing curls. The weights were much, much heavier than I usually use. After Meyrick was done I was asked to pick them up and do some curls while Meyrick was supposed to cheer me on. I was nervous being on TV and having all of the cameras and lighting around, so it never dawned on me to go get some different, lighter weights until I picked Meyrick's up off the ground. I figured I could probably do 3 or 4. I started doing curls and my arms were burning. I knew I should at least try for ten. The camera was rolling and I was down to my last one when the director called out to Meyrick to give me a countdown. In my head I was screaming, "you have to be kidding. Meyrick is going to count me down from 3?!?! I can't do 3." Instead of counting me down from 3 Meyrick started at 6! The camera was still rolling and there was no way I was quitting. I finished the curls and a few minutes later, Meyrick and I were talking about something else when I started to give him hell for counting me down from 6. He bursts out laughing saying that he couldn't believe I completed the curls. He commented that he picked weights that were heavier than usual for himself, because if he was going to be seen on TV lifting weights, they sure as hell had to be impressive. Unfortunately for him, he was never seen on TV lifting those weights as that particular scene was cut and never shown.

I have had so many experiences learning that I could do more than I thought I could. If ever you are working out with a friend who is fitter than you and is willing to push you or if you get to work out with a good personal trainer, you will learn this lesson. Fit people are never surprised to see you dig so deep. They expect it, both of themselves and of you.

Lesson #9: Working Like A Fit Person

The first step in working like a fit person is knowing how hard you are working. Thankfully there is a universal way of measuring how hard a person is working and we will intruduce it in this chapter and show you how to use it to maximize your workouts.

This chapter will also introduce to you the value of hiring a personal trainer, if only occasionally, so that you can learn from an expert how hard you can truly work.

I will then explain how to fuel yourself for a training session and finally, I will impart to you many of the tips and tricks that I have learned from the fittest people I know.

You Have To Know How Hard You Are Working

Although a fit person doesn't have the same problems answering that question as you do (their answer is typically very hard), it is still a very important issue in training, and more so for us. After all, measuring and monitoring improvement is one of the only things that keeps us coming back. I had never thought about measuring how hard I worked out until I had read 'The Body Sculpting Bible for Men'. In it, they had a 'perceived exertion scale' that had you judge how hard you are working on a scale from 1 to 10. I really tried to use this scale, but it was a joke. For an unfit person there is no scale of 1 to 10. There is nothing close. There is a scale of 0 to 1. Zero being doing nothing. 1 being exercising. There was a recommendation that I run at different speeds to get different feelings of exertion as I was running. I tried, I really did, but this was simply impossible. There was 1 speed and 1 measurement. It was several months, after I had completed the couch to 5k program that Meyrick had me work on my second speed. It was still running, but recovering, just like I recovered when walking between running sessions. It was very slow running. It was hardly more than walking, but Meyrick said slow down your running until you are recovering and I found I could do this. Thus I learned my second speed. 2 and 1/2 years later I probably have three or four speeds. Still, I have a very limited scale of exertion with 4 settings: '1. I can keep doing this', '2. I am looking at the clock a lot, so this is definitely time limited', '3. I can do anything for one minute (I tell myself this when it looks like I can't do something for even that long', and '4. Oh My God!!'.

The Heart Rate Monitor

Without self-reporting scales of exertion, how will we measure how hard we are working? We will use a heart rate monitor. Polar is the standard name in heart rate monitors, so I would recommend using one of theirs. The Polar FS3 appears to be an entry level model with all of the bells and whistles you will need. Any decent heart rate monitor will come with a chest telemetry strap. This is the kind you want. Don't go with one that measures your heart rate off of your wrist or finger or whatever else. All that I really need on my heart rate monitor is a stop watch and my heart rate. Mind you, if you are really looking to spend the money and want the best, you will want a Garmin Forerunner 305 (apparently there is a 405 but I have never had the opportunity to use it). I purchased a Forerunner 305 and it is unbelievable. On top of being a heart rate monitor, this watch contains its own GPS. With this you can tell how far you have run, where you have run if you want to download your workouts onto your computer, at which pace you have run and so on. It is so powerful that I haven't even used half of its features. One feature I love, though, is the virtual trainer. You can set a virtual competitor to run against you, at any pace you want (you can set the time for 5k, or 10k or any distance, or just set a rate such as 4 mph, or 10 kph, and you can watch on your watch as this person gets ahead of you or behind you. You can also see by how many meters this person is ahead or behind you. It is tremendously cool.

Okay, cool gadget discussion out of the way. Heart rate monitor is the necessity, everything else is gravy.

Your heart rate directly correlates to how much blood you are pumping through your body which also correlates to how much oxygen your blood is delivering to your muscles, which correlates to how much oxygen your muscles are using. When your muscles are working they need oxygen to function. The more they function, the more they need oxygen. So, your heart rate directly correlates to how hard your muscles are working. This is important because now we have an objective measure of how hard YOU are working. Two people could run a 1 mile at 6.5 mph. For one, it could be easy, for another very difficult. The heart rate of both of these people would show this. As well, psychologically running 1 mile would be very different for these two people, to one it may be excruciating, and to the other a breeze. So imagine if both those people were you. As you continue to exercise it will get easier and easier to run 1 mile. You will be getting fitter and fitter. You will have to run faster or further to work your body to the same level, and that is why heart rate monitoring can be so valuable (and why it will be doubly valuable for you, because you will be able to monitor your improvement and know how much fitter you are getting).

Heart Rate Zones

As you work out your heart works harder. At different levels of workout, different things are occurring, most importantly in how your body is producing energy to continue whatever you are doing. Your body tries to burn the fuel in your body, that is the food you have eaten and the fats you have stored to power your exercise. This can be done when your heart rate is relatively low. Your body burns stored fats for energy when your exertion level is low. As your exertion picks up, you will burn more of the glucose in your blood stream and less stored fat.

As you increase your activity and your heart rate speeds up, your body is less able to burn food to supply the increasing energy needs and uses stored energy to complete the work you are doing. Your muscles store energy within in the form of glycogen. The use of fats, carbohydrates and proteins as energy require oxygen to be burned for fuel. Use of oxygen as part of the energy process is called an aerobic process. When you can no longer burn enough fuel to meet your exercise needs you move into the anaerobic training zone, and this is where your storage of glycogen comes into play. There are no hard and fast rules for exactly when you move from one of these zones to another, but we have some pretty good ideas of where these zones are and how to calculate them.

Table 9-1: Training Zones based upon percentage of maximum heartrate

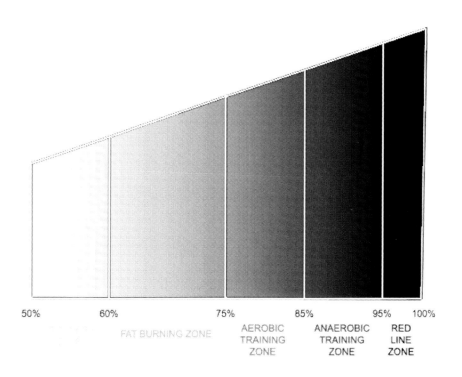

50%	60%		75%	85%	95%	100%
	FAT BURNING ZONE		AEROBIC TRAINING ZONE	ANAEROBIC TRAINING ZONE	RED LINE ZONE	

Calculate Target Heart Rate Zones

Calculating your target heart rate is actually pretty easy. You take the number 220 and subtract your age from it to get your **Maximum Heart Rate** or select your Maximum Heart Rate from the chart below. From there we will calculate our heart rate reserve which will be used to determine our fat burning zone and our aerobic training zone.

Table 9-2: Maximum Heart Rate Based on Age

Age	Maximum Heart Rate	Age	Maximum Heart Rate
60	160	39	181
59	161	38	182
58	162	37	183
57	163	36	184
56	164	35	185
55	165	34	186
54	166	33	187
53	167	32	188
52	168	31	189
51	169	30	190
50	170	29	191
49	171	28	192
48	172	27	193
47	173	26	194
46	174	25	195
45	175	24	196
43	177	23	197
42	178	22	198
41	179	21	199
40	180	20	200

I am 39 years old so my maximum heart rate is 181.

My Maximum Heart Rate - 181

Then to get your **heart rate reserve**, deduct from this number your resting heart rate. Mine is 60. 181-60 = 121. You can measure your resting heart rate before you get out of bed in the morning.

My Heart Rate Reserve = 121

Next calculate your **fat burning training** zone. First calculate the low end of your zone. To do this take 60% of your heart rate reserve and add this number to your resting heart rate. In my example, 60% of 121 is 72 plus 60 is 132. Now calculate the high end. Take 75% of your heart rate reserve and add it to your resting heart rate. 75% of 121 is 91 plus 60 is 151.

My Fat Burning Zone is between 132 and 151

So, I am working out in my fat burning zone when I have a heart rate of between 120 and 151. Yours will probably be slightly different.

Finally, calculate your **Aerobic Training Zone**. The bottom end of the zone is the same 75% of your heart rate reserve added to your resting heart rate. The upper end is 85% of your heart rate reserve. Here my lower end would be 151 and my upper end would be 103 plus 60 or 163.

My Aerobic Training Zone is between 151 and 163

Using your target Heart Rate in Training

So, what is the purpose of all of this work? By using your heart rate, you can actually use an external measure of how hard you are working. When I first saw the fat burning zone and discovered that you really didn't have to work hard to be in this zone, I nearly jumped for joy. I didn't know then, that the whole naming of the zone is tremendously misleading. The idea is that whatever energy you need when working out at this level is generated from the conversion of fat to energy. When you get into the Aerobic Training Zone, you are burning carbohydrates for energy (as you get higher, into the Aerobic/Anaerobic Threshold-80%-90% and Anaerobic Zone 85%-95% you begin using stored glycogen until it is entirely stored energy). The thing is, because you aren't working very hard in the fat burning zone, you aren't burning many calories and therefore you aren't converting much fat to energy. When you ramp up your exercise you actually increase the amount of work you are doing, so even if you are burning carbs and fats, you are still burning more fats when you are working out in the aerobic zone. This is why even though the fat burning zone sounds awesome, it is a bit of a misnomer. What is important here is how many calories you burn and how your body is adapting to burn more energy in the future.

I have spent a lot of time trying to figure out if working out in the fat burning zone will get you leaner or not, but the reality is that is probably won't. The place you want to work out is the aerobic zone. That is where your body will be adapting to improve itself so you can run further and faster. This is where the fit people work out, and so, as with all of our good decisions, this is where we will be working out.

The idea then is that when you are working out, I want you in your aerobic heart rate zone. If you are going on the treadmill or the stairmaster, I want you in your aerobic heart rate zone (most of the machines have the ability to read your Polar telemetry strap-- that is the strap you wear around your heart for your heart rate monitor--and use that to help you calculate your heart rate zone and how long you are in it).

The heart rate monitor will be easy to add into the gym (later in the program), but use it when you are running outside, or climbing stairs or walking as well. This will allow you to take these same principles that will help you get fitter in the gym and let you apply them outside the gym. As well, this will help you understand how your body works when you are really running, like on event day. I did a run recently with an excellent trainer and he had me stay under a 161 heart rate (within my aerobic zone) until the last few miles. It was a 10k run and I got my personal best time by a ridiculous 5 minutes! Looking at the heart rate monitor, knowing I had taken my heart rate up to 184 running up that hill awhile back, I knew that even though I was tired, I wasn't anywhere near worn out. As well, I knew that as long as I was under 161, I really wasn't burning anything up, all of my energy consumption was replaceable. This is opposed to the stored glycogen because there is only so much available. By paying attention to your heart rate, you can makes sure you don't use your stored energy until the end of the race, maximizing your performance. The heart rate monitor is a must have and I highly recommend it to keep your head straight while training and at events, so you can get the most out of yourself.

Personal Trainer

A personal trainer is an expert in resistance training (for the sake of our discussion-many personal trainers also have very deep educations in fitness and nutrition). Ideally a personal trainer will know all about you before your session and will tailor a session to your needs. This is more typical in a boutique gym where most of your visits are with personal trainers. In my gym, I have had two trainers for awhile and they keep track of my fitness levels in their computer. When I get in there, they have a session pre-planned.

Sometimes they write it on a white board to intimidate me. In any case, some things you learn about yourself with these session you cannot learn any other way. The first of these is that "yes", you can. You can do 10 to 15 more repetitions of almost every exercise than you would believe that you can. As soon as you experience this, you will know exactly what I am talking about. Another thing you will learn is that you can pay someone and they can work for you for the money, yet at the same time, they really care about your fitness and will do whatever it takes to help you out. I cannot stress this enough. My trainers have gone out of their way time and time again to help me out. To teach me, to train me. That is the philosophy of my gym, but most people who are into fitness training really want to help you if you want to help yourself. My gym is exceptional. If you have an Innovative Fitness near you, sign up, and go (there is no contract period). It is insanely expensive, but still very much worth it. Everyone I know who goes to a boutique gym says the same thing about theirs, by the way. They swear by them. This is only natural because these gyms understand their clients' needs and work hard to help them achieve their goals.

A personal trainer is a valuable tool to get you where you want to go. They are expensive because you are paying for one on one training. If you have a friend at a similar (or slightly higher) level of fitness, than you can always cut the cost in half and go together (never work out with someone less fit than you unless you are trying to do them a favour).

I cannot recommend enough joining a boutique gym that focuses on personal training and achieving your personal goals, if that is in your price range. I cannot recommend 3 sessions a week with your own personal trainer enough. This is the gold medal package. If you put this together, continue and focus on your out of gym program and work hard in the training sessions, you will undoubtedly succeed. I couldn't afford to do this. I started at 3 sessions a week for a few months, then went down to 2, and then down to 1, increasing back to 2 during the heart of the summer when my training was at its peak, then down to 1 again for the winter. I would go three times if I could. It is that good. If finances aren't an issue for you, I recommend this route. Remember this does not substitute for working hard, not at all, in fact, it requires tremendous work.

Fueling Yourself for a Workout

When you spend so much of your life feeling that food is the enemy, it is strange to turn around and view food as a necessity, but it is. When you start working out, you learn that you can't perform to your best levels unless you have the energy to do so. The way you get this energy is the same way you have always gotten energy, through food.

You have to eat before a workout to have the energy to workout properly. You need to give the food you have eaten a couple of hours to digest before you workout, so you have to time your eating and your workouts carefully. This may require you adjust your eating schedule on workout days, or that you workout 2 hours after one of your standard meals. Two hours is the perfect amount of time to allow your meal to have digested before working out, but you will have to find out if this is the perfect amount of time **for you**.

What you should typically eat is your standard meal, no changes. If you are eating properly, eating meals based upon the balance of proteins, carbs and fats shown in the previous chapter with the correct number of calories, and eating 4 times a day, you should have no problems. These meals are always right and healthy.

If you fail to eat your meal within 2 hours of your training session, then you will need to make some last minute changes on these days. If you eat too soon before your workout, you will feel sick and may throw up during a rigorous session. At the least you will have a full belly feeling during your session and you will be unable to give your best. To get around this, avoid eating anything that will sit in your stomach. Your best bet is a very light meal an hour before your session. Keep it light--a salad, some nuts, some granola (granola bars), protein bars and yogurt. Things along these lines are relatively quick to digest and should not slow down your training session. Again, this is something that you will work out over time.

When you have to eat under one hour before your workout, you are in the straight carb zone. I recommend a fruit bar. By fruit bar, I mean a 100% pure fruit bar, no sugar added. Sun-Rype has fruit to go and fruitsource bars that are excellent for quick energy. Another alternative that can be taken right up until your training session starts is an energy gel. I have depended on Gu Energy Gels on numerous occasions. I like the Espresso Love flavor (when I say like, I mean I can choke it back without throwing up). Each gel or fruit bar gives you about 45 minutes of energy, so plan to have another if your session lasts longer, or have an energy drink such as Gatorade during the session to keep your energy up.

Energy gels and energy drinks are also very helpful for any exercise session that lasts longer than an hour. When I have run half marathons, I always have a Gu with me to take after 1 hour of running. I always take it right before a water station as well, as these things suck the water out of you. **For an hour session or less, you do not need any additional energy.** Don't even think of adding any quick energy to your diet for hour or shorter workout sessions. The purpose of these is to burn stored energy while maximizing your output. This can all be done with the fuel you have by eating 2 hours before your session. I have seen so many people grab a gatorade at the beginning of their workout, or pop a Gu right before every session. It is foolish to do this. You don't need to and you are just adding calories that you need to burn. Fuel properly by eating healthy meals and you will be fine for you exercise sessions. Drink water as you are working out, not energy drinks.

Final Tips On Working Like A Fit Person

I learned all of this from the hard working trainers at Innovative Fitness who I cannot thank enough for this life lesson. It is valuable beyond the gym. It is invaluable in life.

When you think you are giving your most, you aren't

When you are working your hardest, you aren't. The first thing that I learned about working harder was no matter how crappy you feel, no matter how much you don't want to do your exercise session, be there 5 minutes early, get changed and be ready and warmed up before your session starts. Up until this point, I was always 5 minutes late. After all, I am late to everything I do anyways, and 5 minutes really isn't late. That way I knew that even though I was going to work hard, I wouldn't have to work for a whole hour, at least deep down I did. Until I showed up early, I didn't know how important that extra 10 minutes (being already warmed up gets you another 5 minutes) was. It was like putting in 10% more. It also told everyone that I was serious about what I was doing. I was bringing my A game and I expected everyone else to. Mind you this occurred after I was required to walk on the step mill (the evil stairmaster that looks like a truncated escalator) with a medicine ball over my head for 4x the amount of time I was late each session. That teaches a lesson quickly.

Never say no

Never even think "I can't". Unless there is an injury worry, you don't ever want to question yourself or your trainer or your session. You will get another 10% out of yourself at least, if you believe you can do it. When you are flagging, dig deep down inside and pull out whatever you have. I was very good at leaving nothing on the run course, nothing left in the tank on race day, but I realized I never did this for a training session, yet all of the work that you are doing, all of it, is in the training.

With respect to injuries, make sure your trainer or group leader knows of your past injuries. Make sure you know what kinds of motions are bad for them Never do these motions. Unless you are doing a specific rehab program with a trainer, never do motions that cause you pain or have caused an injury in the past. Work with a physiotherapist to rehab these injuries and follow their direct advice about how hard to work and what motions to do. Discuss your classes, or training programs with them. Discussing these things in advance will make sure that the people you are working out with won't see your lack of involvement as being a slacker. This is really important again because people will respond to you bringing your A game. I know a lot of people who use injury and other reasons to not have to work as hard as they can.

Keep digging deeper

As soon as you are in your session, those initial feelings of not wanting to workout will be gone. Unless you are actually coming down with something, you will want to work out once you are moving. **I have gone to workout maybe 200 times feeling like this is the last thing on earth I want to do, and every single time, 5 minutes in, I am committed and excited(I must tell you though, 2 and 1/2 years into training, I still feel like I don't want to workout in the gym right before my session almost every time).** So, don't worry about your initial feelings going into the gym. Regardless of how you feel before the session, wait until 5 minutes into the session and then look for your reservoirs of energy. Don't fear giving it everything you have. Don't fear puking on the floor. Puking is a sign that you are working. Not puking is a sign that you haven't reached that level yet. As Kevin, one of my faithful trainers, said, puking may take time out of your session, but it is a good stomach muscle workout. I will never forget doing some crazy hill repeat runs with Justine, my most consistent trainer. We got to the **top** of the hill, which I had never done before (coincidentally the same hill that Meyrick made me do hill repeats on at the beginning of my journey) and she had me drop and do push ups. I looked at my heart rate monitor and my heart rate was over my maximum of 182. It was 184. I was feeling panicky. I told Justine this and added for good measure that I was almost 40 and I didn't want to have a heart attack. She looked at me, and said, 'Don't worry, you will pass out long before you have a heart attack, now drop and give me 20'. Of course I did as I was told, but I was thinking that a) apparently the idea of me falling down in the street didn't worry her as much as it did me, and b)I need to look at that waiver I signed when I joined the gym because apparently me dying during a session doesn't worry her. The point is, she wasn't worried. She knew I had a lot more to give. A lot! So do you. This is a mental place you need to be in. You have to really want to work out, you have to want the pain, you have to need to know just how deep you can go. If you follow my advice on this, you will see the respect in the eyes of trainers, friends and all who see you workout and hear it directly from their mouths.

Stay to the end, and then some

Never quit during a workout or a session. By workout or session, this could be anything from a planned training session or run, a gym workout or a session with a personal trainer. If you give it all you have and have nothing left before the end, fine, but I doubt this will happen twice. The body adapts very quickly. If you really blow your load and have nothing left one week, then you will probably be able to go 10% to 20% further the next week, and then you will reach the end of your session. What I am saying is don't let it happen twice, and if it happens at all, you had better have amazed everyone with your effort before it happened. If you are running out of energy before the end of a session it is probably a nutrition thing (see nutrition for training sessions in the next chapter). If you can, make a habit of spending 30 minutes on the treadmill after your workout or training session or 30 minutes on a bike. After all, if your heart rate was up that whole time, another 30 minutes of raised heart rate is going to have a profound effect on your weight loss. If your fitness is going to go to the next level as well, your out of gym training session may move past the one hour point in any case, so you will want to get more than one hour in the gym as well.

Here is a tip I learned from *Commando Workout: 4 Weeks to Total Fitness*. My wife bought me this book and recommended I use it. I read it and was thoroughly impressed with the program. It was using this book that I tried to run, tremendously unsuccessfully, the first 10 times or so. The facts and exercise programs in this book are excellent, and if you are going to work out in the gym without a trainer, this is the book to use. I cannot recommend it enough. The use of supersets and cardio-resistance training is exactly what you could use. This is very advanced stuff and will probably produce some tremendous results at this stage. The problem for me was it wasn't going to produce any results from me in my early stages, unless frustration is a result , because I couldn't get there from where I was.

What stuck with me from this book was the pages on exercise visualization. I have since seen and heard this same advice in many different forms in regard to exercising. When you are doing an exercise, you should know the muscle groups you are working out and the correct form. You should then focus on the muscles being worked out and feel them contracting. This process, the process of focusing on your exercise, will produce improved results in your muscles. By the way, the guy who wrote the Commando Workout is a serious expert. He is exactly who you should rely on to help you sculpt your body. He is fit and he has a great program to get you fit. I don't know for sure (and I would hate to anger him), but I am pretty sure that he has always been a fit person.

Action Plan

1. Calculate your target heart rate zones.

2. Get a heart rate monitor and use it.

3. Revise your eating and training schedules until they mesh.

4. Change your attitude about working out. Step it up. Be early, start with 5 minutes always. Stay late, swim a

few more laps, hop on the bike at the end of a weight session. Whatever you are doing, do some more.

5.   Remember, it is in the training that all of the work is being done, not the events. Train like the person you are becoming.

Biggest Difference #9: Motivation Gap

When I was in University, I took a fair amount of psychology courses and in the first one, I learned that there was a concept called cognitive dissonance. I thought it meant, the horrible personal feeling when there was a gap between knowing a wrong behavior and not having the motivation to change it. I later learned it didn't mean this at all (I wasn't all that diligent in studying, actually that was the 'cognitive dissonance' I suffered from all through University), but it was too late, and forever more, to me, cognitive dissonance will always mean feeling terrible because what I am doing is wrong, but not feeling bad enough to do anything to change it. Whatever you call it (feel free to call it by a better name such as Motivational Gap) this idea is very important to understanding some of the obstacles we have in weight loss. **A fundamental difference between fit people and unfit people is the size of the Motivation Gap**. Fit people do not need a lot of knowledge about what they are doing being wrong. As soon as they realize this, they act to eliminate the bad feeling it causes. Unfit people can spend months, years, decades even, with that nagging voice telling them all the reasons why they should change their behavior and that other voice-the one that usually calls the shots, telling them, don't worry it isn't that bad, there is always tomorrow...

Chapter 10
Obstacles

Walls are not there to keep you out, they are there to make you show how much you want it. -Randy Pausch

Make no mistake, no one, and least of all me, said this was going to be easy. But this is doable. It is relatively straight forward. Even so, there are a number of obstacles that we may all have. Some of us will have all of them, some of us only a few, but judging from where we are in our lives, all of us have had some. I am going to list some of the most common obstacles to achieving our goals here, with some suggestions for how to overcome them. In the end though, you have to decide that you aren't going to let these obstacles, or any other, stop you in becoming the you that you want to be. Do you want this enough? Can you climb above these walls?

A Little Background

After I started getting fit, everyone and everything stood in my way. I decided to sign up at a gym with a personal trainer after I had gotten started. This was very expensive and I really had a hard time justifying it, and I was constantly being forced to justify it to my wife. We had two children who I was (and am) very involved with, ages 4 and 6 who ate up all of my free time (being a parent of 2 girls aged 5 and 7, I am fully aware how ironic the term free time is). Still, I had this one opportunity.

I don't know why I took it, I normally wouldn't. I would back down from the pressure, from the constant fighting and tension. That is just what I do. Still, this time I didn't. I don't know if I knew how badly I needed this, deep down. I don't know if I was aware of just how good this group of trainers was, subconsciously. I think, in retrospect, I needed to have someone in my corner. I really needed some support.

One of the things I learned from this was that paid--for support, support for hire, is very effective support. Just because you are paying for it, doesn't make it inauthentic. The people at your gym, especially the trainers will really care about how you do. They are generally fit people and they, like the Borg, want to assimilate you. I think they are equal parts scared of us unfit people and repulsed by us, so when we get fit, we solve that uncomfortable situation for them.

The other more important thing I learned was that until I was willing to put myself first and determine what was important for me, I was never going to be able to get fit. Other people put demands on me all the time; that is what they do. That is their job and they do it well. It is my job to be clear on what I need and want. Nobody is going to do this for me, and nobody is going to do this for you. You aren't doing anyone any favors not taking your life by the reigns, and driving it in the direction that you want to go.

Over time I was able to reduce the number of times I used a personal trainer as my routine became more solidified, until I was able to do this alone. That said, if you can afford a personal trainer, hire one. It is the best money you will spend; just remember, you still need to do the work. The trainer won't do it for you.

213 I YOU ARE NOT A FIT PERSON...

Law of fit people #10
You need to be selfish to get what you want.

Fit people put themselves first. They are much more likely to understand the concept that you put your own oxygen mask on first, and then tend to everyone else. It is a simple concept, but unfit people tend not to get it. So often you see people suffering from debilitating depression, unable to function in the family, and when asked why they don't take care of themselves and get better so they can help their family, they respond that their family comes first and they can't take the time for themselves. Put yourself first and set up the time to make sure your physical needs are met.

It seems wrong to be selfish, but selfishness shouldn't be viewed as a bad thing. By selfishness I mean the simple acts of self awareness and self preservation. To be sure, people can take license with selfishness and even people who don't take care of their physical selves can be demandingly selfish in other ways. If you don't take care of yourself first and foremost, nobody else will. Do not use the excuse of work or family to neglect your physical self. It doesn't make sense and it is only an excuse. If you don't take care of your physical self you will not be able to help your family. You may feel that you are, but you will resent your weight gain and you will blame your loved ones for it. You will have less energy and be less able to be physically active. You won't be able to play with your children in a way that will prepare them for their lives, for their active needs and for their physical tests in life. You will be humiliated by your physical shape and you will show this to the world and your children will learn these feelings and behaviors. They will learn from you and they will inherit your poor relationship with food and your inactive lifestyle.

So, is that being unselfish? Really, if you weigh the outcomes from not setting up time for yourself to get fit, you realize that getting fit and staying fit is a gift for your family. It isn't a question of selfishness really, just a question of showing people, especially the people you love, how to care for yourself.

Lesson # 10: The Obstacles

Families - diet

This here can be a deal killer. If the rest of your family is eating crap, it makes it very very hard to avoid all of this bad food. In ideal cases you control the nutrition in your family. If you do, put your foot down on the really bad foods, and help your family out, or slowly reduce the collection of crap food, starting with the ones that are hardest for you to resist. Also, make sure good choices are around, even if you can't eliminate any of the bad choices. If you feel very strongly about this, sit them down and get them to join you in your quest. It is up to you to convince them of the importance of this journey for you. Realistically you are going to have 1000 times harder of an experience if you can't get the bad food out of your house.

Your other worst case scenario is if your partner eats poorly, refuses to change their habits, and expects you to continue preparing bad foods, or continues preparing bad foods for you. My advice for this is that you have to get your family aligned with your thinking and eating. Look through the recipes and see what you can make that is healthy and will not upset your partner. See if you can get his or her support. This is a tough one. I can recommend the book, *Getting Past No*. It has some awesome strategies for getting agreement in situations where agreement appears impossible. Solutions will require compromise though, so be prepared for that. Find ways to get agreement with your family. I let my kids know that I want to be healthy and I want to live a long time and to do that I have to avoid junk food. I tell them I need their help (and I do). I ask them to look out for me (and they do). I cook a bunch of meals on Sunday when I am home and those are in the fridge and the freezer for the week. Find ways to start down this road, just simple steps, and see if you can build from there. One thing I want to point out here though, is if you have kids and they are eating this crap food, you need to step up and help them kick the habit before they are suffering from a lifelong addiction to bad foods, and a dearth of knowing how to make good choices. It is never easy, so step up and pull off that band aid. Do it for them more so than even yourself.

Friends and Family – attitude

Speaking personally, no one really wanted to see me succeed at my goals. That is, no one until I discovered my friend Meyrick was very supportive. He was tremendously helpful and got me started on a road I never would have followed had he not taken me by the hand and dragged me along it until I found my own way. We don't all have a Meyrick, but you all have me. I am cheering for you. I am you. I am showing you the way. I am taking your hand and dragging you down this path. If you need help/advice, you can email me. Depending on volume of email, I will personally try to answer any question and send out a cheer of support if that is at all humanly possible.

My wife was my biggest anti-supporter. She really didn't want me to succeed. When I would tell people, they would be confused and wonder, 'Isn't she the most likely to benefit from a thinner, fitter you?'. And although that seems true, it really isn't. The people in your life are used to you being who you are. They are made comfortable by the fact that you are overweight. That you clearly don't care how you look. It makes them feel better about themselves and less worried about improving themselves to keep your interest. You are threatening the balance of their whole life. This goes for your brother and sister, your partner, your friends. If they are overweight it is doubly difficult. They will put up obstacles to you. They will laugh derisively and suggest that you 'won't be able to keep this up'. This is where you can draw strength. Don't be hurt by this; it is human nature. Feed off of it. Show them. I doubt I would have achieved my goals had I not had the desire to show my wife how wrong she was about me. The funny thing is, they will come around. They will support you in the end. They will because everyone wants to be associated with a winner, and as you get closer and closer to your goal, as you stick to your plans, day in and day out, as they see the confidence in your eyes as you rack up personal achievement after personal achievement, they will come on board and they will cheer for you, and tell everyone they know about your success. They might even want to join you, and they will want help finding the path, and being dragged down it. This is your chance to give back, like Meyrick did to me, and I am trying to do with you and I hope you jump on this chance and take the time out of your busy schedule to help them. When you have done this, you will know what you have achieved and you will know the measure of yourself was never your body weight, it was the person you wanted to be and the person you have worked so hard to become.

Remember as well, some of your relationships won't be your typical supportive relationships. My brother and I have one of those. We rib each other, we compete at everything and we are best friends, so obviously we don't exactly support each other in a traditional way. That said, nothing, not one single thing, has given me as good a feeling as when I was leaving the transition zone in my first triathlon at about 7 am on a Sunday and I hear, 'Hey Mark' and I see my brother with his hand out for a high five at the fence. He showed up there of his own accord and he stuck around until the end of the triathlon. We talked and laughed and he listened to my stupid stories and then we went for a coffee. I felt like I was part of a team. So don't assume that the only support is someone who helps you or gives you positive reinforcement all of the time. This just isn't realistic. Look for the kind actions within your relationship dynamics and use these items as they are intended, as support.

Budgets

Healthy food, gyms, trainers, race entries, these things are expensive. They are, but each one of these things you put more money into, the easier success may be. That said, no part of this is easy, and some obstacles just increase your determination. If this is you, and your budget is your limiting factor, then you are going to have to take a grim determination in the knowledge that celebrities, with all the money in the world, with personal trainers and chefs and dietitians, don't always succeed, but you are going to. The good news is that running is free. The only cost is the shoes (having good running shoes that work well for your feet is very important. You can find great advice in picking shoes at: http://www.therunningadvisor.com/running_shoes.html), but aside from that all you need is somewhere to run. Gym memberships are remarkably affordable. When you work out the amount of time you are going to be spending in them, now that you have a plan to stick to, the actual cost per visit is quite small. If you would have rented a movie, or eaten a snack, or shopped for something, or grabbed a beer after work, you may actually be saving money, and most gyms provide a safe environment (see picking a gym under fitness). As well, eating less food is actually cheaper than eating more food. That said, nothing is as cheap as fast food in North America. Unhealthy food is cheap. Still, here are some tips for getting some very affordable healthy solutions. And remember, eating less food, not drinking pop, reducing your alcohol consumption, and other healthy decisions really will result in more money in your pocket, not less. As for race entries, join races that allow you to raise money for a cause (discussed in Fitness). These tend to have very inexpensive entry costs and you get to make a difference in the world. As well, after you run a number of events, you can ghost run. Nobody stops people from running events without signing up and getting a number. Keep the time on your stop watch and run along if you can't afford to participate. As well, talk to the race organizer (find his or her name online) and discuss your limited budget. Typically if there is room in the race, and you are willing to forgo the race shirt (or whatever goody they include with the race), you can enter for very little money.

Time

This is the killer for almost everyone. This one may be nearly insurmountable. No matter what, the increased exercise that you will be required to do will be felt in your life if you are too busy already. You probably don't have the time to get everything you need done in a day as it is. If you have kids, that is almost guaranteed. The key is the amount of time you spend training each time will be remarkably limited. It will almost always be an hour or less. You can find an hour 6 days a week. Prepare your lunch and eat it on the way to the gym. Make sure your gym is close to your work or house or both. If it isn't close to both, have a spot near work where you can run, or swim, or go to another gym. Planning here is the key. You are going to have to use your time more efficiently. Almost everyone gets an hour for lunch. See if you can arrive 15 minutes earlier or leave 15 minutes later and get in the whole hour for exercise.

You are much more likely to keep your date with exercise if it is first thing in the morning. If you are at all a morning person, or could possibly become one (again, fit people are almost always morning people, so I am guessing odds are you aren't), then getting up early, before the house is stirring is a great way to get your training in. By getting out of the house before people are awake, you will cut your morning rituals in as much as half. You don't have to talk to anyone, find the kids lunch bags, etc. You just get up and go to the gym or go for a run. As well, you can shower at the gym or sometimes at your work (if you are lucky).

Another option is to cycle to work if that would work for you.

If you have young kids, most gyms have daycare. Make sure the gym that you are using does. If the kids cry and whine about going, tell them you are getting fitter and you need to get fitter to play with them more. I told my kids that they were going to the gym when I was. They thought the day care at the gym was a gym for kids. They loved it, they thought we were all getting a workout. Long after I stopped going to that gym, the kids kept getting me to go back there to work out. Whatever it is that you are doing to get that hour, the key is to schedule the time in advance, like a very important meeting at work, or with your child's teacher. You would never think of missing that appointment or being late for it. Never, ever miss your appointment with exercise. Never. There is a section in Exercise on workouts you can do in your home with no equipment, and some equipment recommendations. These aren't easy as you are likely to get bored, but they are better than nothing and maybe they will make a good punishment if you miss your window at the gym.

Most tracks have large grass infields. If your kids are old enough, you can bring a frisbee, a soccer ball, or other play item and plop your kids in the middle of the field as you run laps. As well, they will get to see you getting fitter and they might be inspired to join you. Another option with kids is to exercise with friends and split the cost of baby-sitting, or alternate who will do the baby-sitting. One thing my friend and I did was to bring the kids to the pool and one parent would watch them while the other swam lengths. Everyone had a great time and we got fitter.

Another thing to think about is that eating healthy and preparing healthy meals is relatively easy and it may buy you some time to exercise. After all, most meals can be eaten over 2 or 3 days (especially with reduced portion sizes), reducing the amount of time you have to prepare them. This time could be time spent getting fit. Fit people always keep their date with exercise. They consider it more important than anything. This is another of the big differences I have seen between fit people and unfit people. The fit people would never think of staying up late and having another drink if they had a run the next morning. Never. You will never be that diligent, so you will have to work harder, that is all.

Finally, chart out your days. Spend a few minutes writing down what you do all day as you do it. Can you rearrange anything? Can you eliminate less healthy activities? Can you do something more efficiently?

If after all of this, you know you have not even 30 minutes a day, no matter how you rearrange your life, then you are going to have to make some serious adjustments to your lifestyle. You can still eat better, and the exercise may have to wait. You don't want to be burning the candle at both ends for too long if there is any chance you can avoid it though. The stress will get to you. So, while you try to adjust your lifestyle so you can incorporate exercise, eat healthy and remember that this, too, shall pass.

Injury

Injury will get us all. It is just a likelihood. I didn't think much about it when I started exercising and I don't expect you to think much about it either, until it happens to you.

My number one strategy for injury was to take up swimming. It worked. While I was resting my knees from Patella Femoral (a very common-for beginners-and potentially serious injury where the cartilage in the back of your kneecaps loses its structural strength, resulting in inflammation and pain) I swam. I had taken up swimming way earlier because I knew I wasn't starting this exercise thing in my youth. I knew I was going to have problems down the road and I couldn't lose the forward momentum that I had.

In any case, having a back up exercise or 2 or 3 is a good idea. If you injure yourself running, it is good to know you can switch to the pool and to a lesser extent the bike, and that is what I did.

So, if you become injured, consult your doctor, and your physiotherapist. Listen to them. Don't try to do anything that they tell you not to do. Take it easy and rest your body. At this point in your exercise, that is probably the last thing that you want to do, but you will have to. This injury does risk sidelining your fitness goals to be sure, but you don't want to risk sidelining your future fitness entirely. This can happen.

Try to find ways to keep active with exercises that don't use the part of your body that you have injured. If you can't even do that, than take it easy, continue to eat better and wait. When you are ready, take the number of months that you have taken off, multiply it by 4 minus the number of years you have been training (for example if you have been training for 3 or more years, multiply it by one, 2 years, multiply the months by 2, and one year, multiply the months by 3 (and by one year I mean you are in your first year of training). Go back that far in your training schedule and start there. So, if you are injured for 3 months and you are in your first year, go back 9 months in your training schedule. What were you doing 9 months ago? Start at that part in your physical training schedule this time out.

If you are having a hard time resting and taking it easy, take joy in realizing that the old you would have loved to have rested, in fact that was all it did. Take this energy and desire to get back out there and remember it when you get that chance again.

Holidays and Celebrations

Don't sweat the holidays and celebrations. Sure, if they happen all the time, or a major holiday like Christmas is coming up right as you are starting the program, then you may have a problem. Otherwise, the odd holiday will just be a period you need to get over. Here are some tips.

1.   Plan a holiday workout schedule. You may have your work or everyday workout schedule down. Nothing will destroy this faster than a holiday break. You will need to commit to new, more flexible times to work out. Plan them in advance and post them in the kitchen or wherever your family will see them. Discuss your schedule with them in advance so that nothing will stand in the way of you getting your workout in. Again, keep your date with fitness. That is non-negotiable.

2.   When traveling, make sure your hotel has a workout room. If you are traveling with friends of the family, this is a

great chance to get your friends involved with you in running or exercising or whatever.

3.   You know what the good food choices are now, so make them as much as possible.   Despite your good intentions, you will probably eat a bit more crap than you want and then you will discover what I did this Christmas-the cravings come back with a vengeance. I had to re-kick my sugar habit after Christmas and it was as hard as anything I have done. A few days later though, I am fine again and eating well, but there was a terrifying moment of believing that I had lost control. I didn't feel the sense of control when I was eating properly and had all of my meal plans in place. Again, don't worry, just put one day in the books with a good meal plan acted on, and then another and so on. You will be right back in control in no time. I did have to consume a few more calories to get my control back and I couldn't have fit more fruit in my fridge if I had tried, but in the end, I got back very quickly and I didn't even notice much of a spike on the scale. I had poorly planned my exercise schedule over the holidays as well, so it wasn't until I was exercising properly that I really felt all my control come back, so stick to the schedule.

Action Plan

This action plan is very simple. Solve your problems. They are yours, take ownership, make a plan and take the action necessary to get the obstacle out of your way. Surmount it or sidestep it, I don't care, but get beyond the obstacle. You can do this.

Biggest Difference #10: Excuses

We see excuses as reasons to not do things. Fit people see excuses as things that need changed to make their lives work. I remember in University some teacher telling me that my reason why I didn't get my work done was just an excuse. I remember thinking, no, it is actually the *reason* I didn't get my work done (I have no idea if it was true or not, but I know it was compelling because true or not I would have embellished it until it was compelling). I have never been able to communicate well with people who have the attitude that a reason why you failed to achieve something is just an excuse.

That was until I started to succeed at tough goals such as fitness. Then I started to notice people telling me the same reasons for why they were unable to get fit. Reasons that I had used and, it appeared, that everyone uses. These were preventable reasons, they were foreseeable and avoidable. I realized then that I was thinking, 'but you knew that would happen and you didn't do anything to prevent it, so really that isn't a reason, that is an excuse'. I would say to them, 'Okay, that sounds bad, but now you know it can happen, how are you going to make sure it won't happen again?' Of course, they wouldn't.

No obstacle is insurmountable, once you know what it is. Do you want it bad enough? Whenever I have an obstacle I think of Randy Pausch and I think, is this wall designed to keep me out, or just show how much I want it?

Take what were your excuses and write them down. They are very important. Don't run from them, and don't minimize them. Therein lie the answers to your fitness. Solve those problems, tackle them, take them on and you can be fit.

It was this realization, that all of the excuses that I currently had in life were actually lessons waiting to be learned, that I knew I was going to be fit for life. These were pointers to solutions. Fit people know that if there is an obstacle, a reason for not being able to achieve something, then you have to change your plan to go around it, or work harder to go over it. An excuse is just knowledge of something that has to change. Of course when I realized I was beginning to think like a fit person, I began to be afraid...very afraid.

Chapter 11
Recipes

A good cook is a certain slow poisoner, if you are not temperate.
~Voltaire

I have broken down the recipes into breakfast, lunch, supper and dinner. For all intents and purposes all of these meals are interchangeable. I quite often eat the oatmeal once in day, even if it is for dinner. I am terrible on the organization, but I always have oatmeal fixings, so it is good to go when I haven't planned ahead. I have chosen these recipes because they are go-to meals, that is they are likely to make it into your standard weekly rotation. More importantly I have chosen them because they are **easy**. Finally, these are meals that although healthy, aren't 'fit person' healthy, full of mung beans, chick peas and lentils. They are tasty for everyone, even kids.

Each of the items is organized as a meal or recommendations for full meals are given. Unless otherwise stated each recipe is for a single serving. I have also included 3 sauces for dipping, tzaziki, raita and healthy ranch. These sauces, when made at home with no-fat yogurt are low calorie, low fat and full of cooling flavor. Some of these meals are begging for a little cooling.

BREAKFAST

When grilling vegetables, spray some Pam© spray into the non-stick skillet. I always use nonstick as it reduces the amount of oil that you need to use to cook with. Mix and match these meals. When you see any meat, you can switch it with the same amount of any other meat. Add as many vegetables as you like and mix and match them as you see fit.

THIS IS THE MOST IMPORTANT BREAKFAST MEAL THAT I HAVE. THIS ONE MEAL ALONE HAS PROBABLY BEEN MORE RESPONSIBLE FOR MY WEIGHT LOSS THAN ANY OTHER. YOU HAVE TO EAT BREAKFAST AND THIS ONE IS WELL BALANCED, EASY TO MAKE AND KEEPS YOU FULL WELL INTO THE DAY.

Easy Oatmeal & Ham

1/3 cup large flake oatmeal	2/3 cup water
10 blueberries	1/4 cup All Bran Buds©
1 Tbsp granola	1/4 cup of milk
2 oz (50 grams) black forest deli ham (about 3 slices)	

1. Put the oatmeal flakes in a bowl with the water and half of the blueberries.
2. Microwave for 4 and 1/2 minutes.
3. Add the remaining 5 blueberries stir the oatmeal and bury the blueberries so they will warm up.
4. Add granola, All Bran Buds© and milk when you are ready to eat.
5. Place the black forest ham in a non-stick frying pan and fry for a minute or so on high heat..
6. Serve

Final thoughts: I normally keep a bag of frozen blueberries in the freezer for this meal, but I often use fresh blueberries when they are in season. They both work equally well. The blueberries added at the beginning dissolve into the oatmeal and give it a great overall flavor. The final blueberries get hot, like blueberries in pancakes and they taste fantastic. Ten is just a suggestion as to how many to add, modify this number for what works for you. You can also add cut up pieces of strawberries, peaches or raspberries if you like.

Modify this recipe to make it work for you. You can add raisins or other fruit. You don't have to add the granola, but don't add any sugar. This breakfast doesn't need any.

I like black forest ham, but there are many different varieties at the deli, including non-fat and honey ham. You can also cook up turkey or roast beef if you want. Choose what works for you.

THIS IS THE RUSH BREAKFAST MEAL. WHEN YOU ONLY HAVE A MINUTE OR TWO IN THE MORNING BUT YOU STILL WANT A MEAL, THIS IS A QUICK ONE.

All Bran Buds Cereal & Yogurt

1 cup skim milk	1 100 gram activia yogurt
1/3 cup All Bran Buds©	

1. Mix everything in a bowl and serve.

Final thoughts: I like activia yogurt, but you can add any type of yogurt you like. One 100 gram container of activia contains 100 calories. You can have up to 200 calories of yogurt with this meal, so choose 200 calories of your favorite. As well, choose the flavor you like. I like strawberry and vanilla, but this is entirely up to you.

You can add as much cut up fresh fruit as you like to this breakfast.

This meal is a little light on protein, so you can always eat a slice of ham or turkey with it or a link of turkey sausage.

THIS WAS THE FIRST BREAKFAST OUT OF THE ZONE DIET THAT I ATE. IT IS A GREAT WEEKEND BREAKFAST WITH A CUP OF COFFEE ON A SUNNY MORNING SITTING ON A PATIO.

Smoked Salmon on a Bagel

---

4 oz. smoked salmon

2 Tbsp low fat cream cheese

1 Weight Watchers© whole wheat bagel

---

1. Spread cream cheese on bagels, place smoked salmon on top and serve as 2 open faced halves.

Final thoughts: You need to be very careful about what bagel you use here. If you are a traditionalist and know what bagels are supposed to taste like (they don't taste like store-bought by the way), then when you cut your bagel, slice it into three slices and throw away the middle slice. You can also serve this on bread or toast as well.

If you like your bagel toasted, you can do that as well.

Some people like onions and capers on their smoked salmon. If you do feel free to add them. As well you could add a tomato slice to this sandwich.

THIS IS A VERY HEALTHY, VERY FILLING MEAL. IF I HAVE SOME TIME OR IF I HAVE THE RIGHT LEFT OVERS IN THE FRIDGE, THIS IS THE BEST WEEKEND BREAKFAST THAT I CAN THINK OF.

Denver Omelette

2 links turkey sausage	1 egg
4 Tbsp egg white	1 oz cheese
1 onion	1 pepper (green or yellow)
salt	pepper
1 slice of Weight Watchers© whole wheat toast	

1. Cook turkey sausage links before starting omelette. Dice one of the sausage links.
2. Grate or crumble your cheese. Slice your vegetables.
3. Whip egg with egg whites until mixed and add salt and pepper to liking.
4. Fry up onions and peppers on high heat until cooked to your liking, about 5 minutes.
5. Transfer vegetables to a side plate and turn the heat to medium low.
6. Pour eggs into frying pan and cook until bottom is cooked and top is slightly runny.
7. Add the vegetables, cheese and 1 diced turkey sausage link evenly to the cooking eggs.

8. Flip one half of the eggs over the other to seal up the omelette.
9. Serve with one turkey link and 1 piece of whole wheat toast.

Final thoughts: If you don't have any of the turkey links or don't want to bother cooking them up, you can use shredded deli ham. Take 2 slices, fry them both and then shred one and add it to the omelette.

I know that egg white omelets are very healthy, but I cannot live without at least one egg yolk in there. I find this blend of essentially 1 egg to 2 egg whites to be a very workable ratio. If this doesn't work for you, start with 2 egg to 1 white and slowly transition.

Cheese is a very important decision here, mostly because there isn't a lot. A dream omelette has so much cheese you can hardly find the eggs in it, but that is so unhealthy it is ridiculous. I have found that 1 oz of cheese is more than enough cheese to get the flavor you need. What I have discovered though is that the sharper cheeses are so much better when you don't have a lot of cheese. They pack a ton of flavor into a small bite. Ideally I have 1/2 an ounce of feta and 1/2 an ounce old cheddar. Because I eat less cheese nowadays, I treat myself to aged 10 year old cheddar whenever I can.

I don't love mushrooms so I didn't add them to this omelette, but if you like mushrooms, you can either fry them with the vegetables or add them uncooked to the omelette right before you fllp.

I highly recommend adding diced tomatoes. If you like you can add green onions, asparagus or cauliflower.

All of this food is still just one serving. Just double, triple or quadruple up the ingredients to serve 2,3 or 4 people. You can make separate omelets in a small frying pan or one large omelette in a larger frying pan.

This meal can be so easy to prepare if you have cooked up the sausage links earlier in the week and slowly doled

them out. As well, if you have prepared the grilled onions
and peppers on the barbecue and have some left over,
you pretty much have this meal ready to go. Nothing
tastes better than the grilled vegetables the next morning
in an omelette.

I HATE TO ADMIT HOW OFTEN I DEPEND ON THIS QUICK BREAKFAST. IT IS QUICK AND EASY AND WILL GUARANTEE THAT YOU GET A HEALTHY START TO YOUR DAY. NOBODY IS EVERY TOO RUSHED TO EAT THIS FOR BREAKFAST. AS WELL, A LARGE CONTAINER OF PROTEIN SHAKE POWDER APPEARS QUITE EXPENSIVE, WHEN YOU WORK OUT HOW MANY SERVINGS IT HAS, IT IS A VERY COST EFFECTIVE MEAL.

Protein Shake & Fruit

1 scoop protein powder	1 cup skim milk or water
4 ice cubes	1 cup mixed fruit

1. Put protein powder, milk or water and ice cubes into a blender and mix.
2. Serve in a glass.

Final thoughts: I cannot recommend enough getting a Magic Bullet© for protein shakes. I just throw all of the ingredients in the cup, screw on the top and blend for 10 seconds. You can drink the shake right out of the mixer cup.

Choose whatever flavor and brand of protein powder you like. I like Sytha-6© Mochachino. One thought though is you could use vanilla flavor and throw your fruits right into the blender/Magic Bullet.

Choose whatever fruit you like, such as an apple or strawberries, or you could substitute a slice of Weight Watchers wheat toast, lightly buttered. I noticed over time that if I didn't have some fruit or toast with my protein shake, I get grumpy. I think I need the carbs just to stay happy.

You can make a shake in a shaker cup as well and take this with you to work or wherever you go. The protein shake can save you so many slips if you prepare yourself well. Keep some scoops of powder with you and a shaker cup. Anywhere there is water you can eat a filling healthy meal.

THIS IS A QUICK WEEKEND BREAKFAST THAT IS QUITE TASTY. I LOVE IT BECAUSE I MISS EGGS ON TOAST FROM TIME TO TIME. THIS ISN'T THE MOST FILLING MEAL EITHER, SO IT IS BEST EATEN WHEN YOU WAKE UP LATE.

Eggs and Ham on Toast

2 eggs	3 slices of ham
1 oz cheese	Salt and Pepper
2 slices Weight Watchers© wheat bread	

1. Toast bread and lightly butter.
2. Poach or fry the eggs to your liking.
3. Fry ham slices.
4. Slice cheese and place on toast.
5. Put ham slices on cheese.
6. Place eggs on top of cheese.
7. Salt and Pepper to taste and serve.

Final thoughts: There really is no vegetable or fruit with this meal so it just isn't that filling. Still it is a great breakfast and it tastes fantastic.

You can add some fried onions and peppers to this sandwich or a slice of tomato on each piece of toast.

LUNCH

I have included some of the lighter
meals here, mostly soups, salads and
sandwiches. All of the meals are
interchangeable though, so feel free to
eat lunch for supper or supper for dinner
or dinner for lunch and so on....

SOUP ISN'T JUST GOOD FOR YOU, IT IS GREAT. IT
FEELS GOOD ON A COLD DAY OR WHEN YOU AREN'T
FEELING GREAT, BUT MUCH MORE IMPORTANTLY, IT IS
SO GOOD FOR YOU. AVOID CREAM SOUPS, BUT
BROTH SOUPS ARE GREAT. YOU CAN MAKE A FRESH
SOUP OR USED CANNED, IT REALLY DOESN'T MATTER.

Soup & Open Face Toasted Sandwich

---

1 can soup

2 oz Cheddar Cheese

2 pieces Weight Watchers© whole wheat bread

---

1. Heat the soup.
2. Slice the cheese, put it on the bread and broil in an oven at 500 degrees for about 4 minutes, until it is cooked the way you like it.
3. Serves 2 people (cut the recipe in half for 1).

Final thoughts: I love Campbell's© Soups. My favorite has always been Vegetable Beef condensed soup (that is the soup you have to add a can of water to). Next favorites are anything in the Chunky© line. I love all of the southwestern soups because they taste like a thin chili. I love chili, but it isn't the healthiest selection. Soup is. One of the go to soups in our family is Chunky Chicken Noodle. Keep a bunch of these soups in your house, they are great to have around the house all of the time and a full can is under 400 calories. The new Chicken Noodle soup is under 250 calories so you can have a whole can of soup to yourself plus the sandwich.

When you are using your own soups, a bowl is a good serving size and should be more than enough for you to eat.

Add onions, tomatoes and/or peppers to the toasted cheese sandwich for a flavor that is out of this world. It takes on a Bruschetta with cheese sort of quality. The open faced toasted cheese sandwich can be modified in so many ways to make it a truly gourmet experience. Herbs and spices can really bring it to life.

I DISCOVERED THIS SALAD AND CHICKEN COMBO AT A RESTAURANT DOWN THIS STREET FROM WHERE I WORK. EVERY FIT PERSON I KNOW WAS TELLING ME HOW GOOD THEIR FOOD WAS, BUT THEY WERE FIT PEOPLE, SO IT WASN'T LIKE I WAS GOING TO LISTEN TO THEM ON MATTERS OF FOOD. TURNS OUT THEY WERE RIGHT.

Mediterranean Salad (& Indian Chicken)

1/4 cup of olive oil	2 cloves garlic
8 celery stalks	2 tomatoes
1 red onion	1 sweet onion
3 peppers (green, yellow and orange)	4 Tbsp fresh squeezed lemon juice
1/2 tsp. salt	4 Tbsp white wine vinegar
1 tbsp fresh cilantro	1tbsp fresh parsley
pepper to taste	

1. Chop up all of the vegetables into bite sized pieces.
2. Finely chop the herbs and mix with the olive oil, salt, pepper, vinegar and lemon juice.
3. Put the vegetables in a large bowl. pour over dressing and mix.
4. Serve

Final Thoughts: This is my favorite salad dressing as it has such a freshness and tartness. This salad tastes better and better the longer it sits, so make it an hour in advance of when you are going to eat it and you can store it for days in the fridge. As always, mix in the vegetables you like. There is no protein in this salad so accompany it with the following chicken dish or 4 oz of any meat. This is an easy lunch to throw in a couple of plastic containers for lunch at work.

I HAD TO FIGURE OUT WHAT WAS IN THE SALAD RECIPE AND MODIFY IT MYSELF BECAUSE THE OWNERS LEFT TOWN, BUT BEFORE THEY DID, THEY TOLD ME HOW THEY MADE THEIR FANTASTIC CHICKEN. THEY GRILLED CHICKEN AND ADDED BOTTLED TANDOORI SAUCE.... THIS RECIPE INCLUDES ALL OF THE INGREDIENTS TO MAKE YOUR OWN SAUCE, BUT IT IS SO EASY TO USE BOTTLED, IF YOU FIND A GOOD ONE. THE BEST ONE I KNOW OF IS NANA'S KITCHEN TANDOORI BBQ SAUCE©.

Spicy Grilled Indian Chicken

4 chicken breast halves	1 tbsp lemon juice
1 tsp olive oil	1/2 cup 0% fat greek yogurt
1 tbsp paprika	1 tbsp tumeric
1 tbsp grated fresh ginger	2 cloves of garlic
1 tsp curry powder	1 tsp coriander
1 tsp chili powder	1 tsp cumin

1. Mix all of the ingredients except the chicken, this is the marinade and the sauce.
2. Split this liquid into 2 parts, one to marinade and one to top. Never use your marinade again on top of cooked foods, it isn't safe.
3. Marinade the chicken for at least 2 hours, preferably overnight.
4. Grill the chicken on an electric grill, in the oven on broil or over the barbecue, until cooked through.

When cooking a slightly crispy brownness is desired on the outside.

5. Let the remaining sauce that was NOT used in the marinade come to room temperature or warm it in the microwave and then divide it in 4 and top each of the pieces of chicken.

6. Serves 4

Final thoughts: This is one of a million grilled chicken recipes. I love marinating my chicken in a teriyaki sauce or soy sauce and then just adding a little of fresh teriyaki or soy after grilling. I also include a greek marinade for a shish kabob recipe on page 204. This marinade works just as well for grilled chicken. Keep experimenting with marinades and flavors.

The heat of the spicy grilled indian chicken really pairs well with the Mediterranean salad though. You can also put a little bit of the raita from page 210 on this chicken to cool it down a little. Note that when you are using greek yogurt, use the plain flavor for making sauces and marinades and use the vanilla yogurt for breakfast and with fruits and cereals.

I LOVE SALAD. I ALWAYS HAVE, BUT TO ME A
SALAD MEANT ICEBERG LETTUCE WITH DRESSING ON IT.
I HAVE SLOWLY ALLOWED IN THE CARROTS,
TOMATOES AND CUCUMBER, AS WELL AS THE OTHER
TYPES OF LETTUCE LEAVES. IF YOU ARE NEW TO
SALADS, DON'T RUSH INTO IT. START WITH A
RELATIVELY PLAIN SALAD AND WORK YOUR WAY UP.

Healthy Salad (& Sliced Steak)

Lettuce	1 tomato
1/2 cucumber	1 carrot
2 tbsp healthy vinaigrette dressing	A small amount of croutons

1. Slice the tomato and cucumber. Slice or grate the carrot
2. Toss vegetables in with lettuce and dressing and toss.
3. Put croutons on top and serve

Final Thoughts: Choose a lettuce blend that contains some variety of greens, including some red cabbage. You can get a primarily iceberg blend if you like, but make sure to have some variety in there. If you don't like vegetables in your salad very much, start out by cutting the vegetables very small. Grate the carrots and cabbage, and dice the tomatoes and cucumbers very small. This makes them so much easier to eat and will help you get used to them in your salad.

A lot of fit people I know also add roasted, unsalted pecans, sunflower seeds, pomegranates, mandarin orange segments, strawberries and dried cranberries. Any and all of these are great additions to a salad.

When you start eating healthier dressings, such as Renee's Gourmet Vinaigrettes©, with no added sugar, they may taste a little bitter to you. Adding the fruits I mentioned earlier or fresh grated carrot to your salad will massively improve the taste. You won't want to eat your salads with sugary dressings after awhile. This meal has no protein in it yet so serve it with the steak on the next page or any 4 ounces of meat.

A GRILLED STEAK IS ONE OF THE MOST PERFECT FOODS ON EARTH, BUT MOST PEOPLE DON'T ASSOCIATE IT WITH A SALAD. I HAVE TO BE HONEST AND SAY I DIDN'T EITHER UNTIL I WAS IN SAN ANTONIO, TEXAS AND WAS SERVED A STEAK SALAD FOR LUNCH. IT WAS INCREDIBLE.

Fire Grilled Sliced Steak

1 8 oz New York Steak	olive oil
course salt	pepper

1. Brush steak with olive oil and pepper.
2. Grill until desired doneness.
3. Let sit for 5 minutes and then salt to taste
4. Slice into thin slices, serves 2.

Final Thoughts: Get used to grilling meat, it is a skill that everyone should have. The Barbecue Bible by Steven Raichlen is a great book to have for anyone who owns a barbecue.

I love a good teriyaki steak as well. To make this steak, just marinate your meat in a good teriyaki sauce the day before you are going to cook it.

Garlic salt is an excellent flavor to put on your steaks as well. Additionally, a great steak rub or seasoning salt tastes great. One of my favorites is Cajun Blackened Steak.

SUPPER/TEA

Typically I am just trying to get from lunch to dinner with this meal, although quite often this is my pre-workout meal, as I exercise after work quite often. Eating this meal at 4 gives me a chance to get it out of my stomach by the time I am exercising. I am going to recommend mostly meal sized snacks here, although once again, these meals are interchangeable.

MY MOM HAS ALWAYS EATEN GREEK SALADS, BUT I AVOIDED THEM LIKE THE PLAGUE. OVER TIME THOUGH, GREEK SALAD HAS BECOME ONE OF MY FAVORITE FOODS. THE SALTINESS OF THE FETA AND THE OLIVES WITH THE POWERFUL FLAVOR OF THE ONIONS AND PEPPERS, ALL DRENCHED IN A SPICY VINAIGRETTE DRESSING.

Greek Salad

2 tomatoes	1 cucumber
1 red onion	8 Kalamata Olives
2 green peppers	4 Tbsp Olive Oil
5 oz. feta cheese	1/4 Tsp. salt
1/4 Tsp. pepper	1 Tbsp dried oregano
2 cloves garlic	2 Tbsp lemon juice

1. Dice the vegetables to the size you would like and put in bowl.
2. Crumble the feta cheese and put in bowl with vegetables.
3. Add the olives, and the dressing and toss thoroughly.
4. Serves 2.

Final Thoughts: This meal is a little high in fat and low in protein, but it is so full of vegetables. You can eat a little less salad and add a little bit of meat to balance out this meal a little better. The calories are in the cheese, oil and olives, so you can reduce any one of these to make this meal a little healthier.

Canned black olives are not Kalamata olives. You can get these olives anywhere and they taste fantastic. They are so full of flavor, they explode in your mouth.

Some feta cheese has a great sharp flavor, but some others have a very creamy mild taste. I like my cheeses with some bite, so I find the driest, sharpest feta I can.

You can get a greek salad at just about any deli counter, so this is a great meal to have when you are out. As well, many pizza places have these salads. Try having one small piece of pizza and a salad instead of multiple pieces of pizza.

THIS IS A GREAT AND SUPER EASY CHICKEN DISH. THIS ONE HAS BEEN IN OUR WEEKLY ROTATION FOR A LONG TIME. THE BEST PART ABOUT THIS CHICKEN IS THAT IT TASTES JUST AS GOOD COLD.

Easy Chicken (& Szechwan Green Beans)

1 full chicken breast(2 halves)	1/4 cup soy sauce
4 tsp olive oil	1/2 lemon
Pinch of rosemary	Pinch of Basil
Pinch of pepper	

1. Slice the chicken into about 30 small slices.
2. Combine all of the ingredients and marinate overnight.
3. Pour the chicken and marinade into a hot frying pan and cook on medium heat with the lid on for 10 minutes, stirring from time to time.
4. Take lid off and turn heat up to high. Cook until all of the liquid absorbs back into the chicken, stirring from time to time.
5. Serves 2.

Final Thoughts: You can use chicken tenders instead of chicken breasts. These make this meal even easier. If you like dark meat you can also throw in some chicken pieces, like thighs and cook them this way as well.

You can try adding some orange juice with the lemon juice or instead to make this meal a little sweater.

This can be used as the 4 ounces of meat in any meal, including the healthy salad. This also means that you can add any number of vegetable dishes to this to fill yourself up, including the szechuan green beans on the next page.

THIS WAS A SIMPLE RECIPE THAT HAS JUST BECOME PART OF OUR FAMILY ROTATION BECAUSE THE KIDS REALLY LIKE IT. I WAS SHOCKED WHEN THEY ACTUALLY REQUESTED IT AND THEY EAT ALL OF THE BEANS, SO I HAVE JUST STUCK WITH IT. THIS VEGETABLE SIDE DISH TASTES GREAT SO GIVE IT A SHOT. BY THE WAY, I HAVE NO IDEA IF THIS HAS ANYTHING TO DO WITH SZECHUAN CUISINE, AS I WENT WITH THE NAME TO IMPRESS THE KIDS.

Szechwan Green Beans

1 pound green beans	1/4 cup soy sauce
1 Tbsp olive oil	1/4 tsp. sesame oil
6 cloves of garlic	1 tsp. fresh ginger (optional)

1. Wash the beans, break off the ends and discard, then cut into 3 inch lengths.
2. steam or boil for about 4 minutes and set aside.
3. In a frying pan fry the garlic and ginger in the olive and sesame oil.
4. Add the soy sauce and green beans to the oil and cook for at least 2 minutes depending on how crispy or soft you want your beans. We cook them for quite awhile until the beans are a little softer.
5. Serve.

Final Thoughts: A pound of green beans will feed at least 4 people, but I don't put serving sizes on vegetables because I encourage you to eat as much as you can. Eat these until you are full if you like.

I don't use the ginger very often because I haven't had much ginger in the house lately. They taste great without the ginger and a little better with the ginger so if you have ginger add it. As well, all foods taste better with alcohol so if you want to step this up to a more gourmet meal, add a splash of chinese cooking wine or Sake if you have some.

You can also add a sprinkle of red pepper flakes to this meal when you fry the garlic.

YOU CAN GET A FRUIT AND YOGURT CUP JUST ABOUT ANYWHERE. THEY ARE A PRETTY GOOD SNACK SO LONG AS THE FRUIT IS FRESH CUT FRUIT AND NOT SERVED IN A SUGARY FRUIT SYRUP. YOU CAN MAKE SURE YOU GET A HEALTHY FRUIT AND YOGURT CUP BY MAKING YOUR OWN. BY USING NON-FAT GREEK YOGURT YOU WILL MAKE A PHENOMENALLY RICH SNACK THAT HAS A FAIR AMOUNT OF PROTEIN.

Greek Yogurt Parfait

10 large sliced strawberries	20 blueberries
1/4 cup of granola	10 raspberries
2 cups vanilla 0% fat Greek Yogurt	1/3 cup All Bran Buds© (optional)

1. Mix the berries and the granola.
2. Add the dry ingredients right before you eat.
3. Serve.

Final Thoughts: Use fruits that you like, these berries are just a suggestion.

2 cups of yogurt are a lot, so you may not want to add a little more granola or the All Bran Buds©. If you prefer to eat your yogurt without granola, by all means go ahead. Granola is just a sweet grain concoction that really isn't good for you and I just add it to food for its texture and great flavor.

You can buy frozen mixed berries and thaw them out in the microwave before adding them to the yogurt, that way you can always be sure you have this snack on hand.

DINNER

Typically I am just trying to get from lunch to dinner with this meal, although quite often this is my pre-workout meal, as I exercise after work quite often. Eating this meal at 4 gives me a chance to get it out of my stomach by the time I am exercising. I am going to recommend mostly meal sized snacks here, although once again, these meals are interchangeable.

I HAVE BEEN MAKING STIR FRIES FOR YEARS. MIND YOU, WHEN I WAS FIRST MAKING THEM, I WOULD PICK THROUGH ALL OF THE VEGETABLES AND JUST EAT THE MEAT.

Stir Fry

1 bag baby carrots	3 cloves garlic
1 onion	1 stalk celery
1 green pepper	1 yellow pepper
1 orange pepper	1 bunch broccoli
1 bunch cauliflower	1 can bamboo shoots
1 can water chestnuts	A handful bean sprouts
2 full breasts of chicken	1/4 soy sauce
A handful of pea pods	1 Tbsp olive oil

1. Slice the chicken into small, bite size strips.
2. Cut the carrots, onion, peppers, cauliflower and broccoli into bite sized pieces.
3. Heat oil in a large wok. Add the onion, garlic and celery and cook them until the onions and garlic are translucent.
4. Add broccoli, cauliflower, carrots, bamboo sprouts, water chestnuts, peppers, and chicken and cook for 5 minutes.
5. Add soy sauce and bean sprouts and put a lid on your wok for 5 more minutes, or until chicken is cooked through.

6. Serves 4 people.

Final Thoughts: Pick vegetables you like. You can always pick around some vegetable you don't like and you will probably come to enjoy them over time, so be daring. This is a chicken stir fry but feel free to use 4 ounces of beef per serving, or fish or pork or whatever meat you choose. You can marinate the meat in the soy sauce as well if you want it to have more flavor.

Vary the times of adding the vegetables based on how crisp you like each of your different vegetables.

I find the soy sauce so easy I don't bother with making a home made teriyaki sauce very often. They taste great. You can also go with a bottled teriyaki sauce if you like the taste.

There are so many great recipes for stir fries out there, keep experimenting. Search the internet or get a good cookbook.

I MODIFIED THIS RECIPE FROM A SKILLET MEAL THAT I DISCOVERED AT A LOCAL CASUAL DINING RESTAURANT, SAMMY J PEPPERS©. THIS IS ONE OF MY FAVORITE HEALTHY RECIPES. THIS IS JUST A SLIGHT VARIATION ON THE STIR-FRY RECIPE ON THE PREVIOUS PAGE. THE VARIATION IS THE KEY TO THIS RECIPE THOUGH. I CRAVE HOT WINGS FROM TIME TO TIME AND THIS MEAL CRUSHES THOSE CRAVINGS. THE BEST PART ABOUT IT THIS RECIPE IS THAT THE VEGETABLES ABSORB MORE OF THE HOT SAUCE THAN THE MEAT, SO THEY BECOME THE STARS!

Hot Sauce Skillet

2 Tbsp vegetable oil	Tbsp Hot Sauce
1/4 cup soy sauce	1/2 chicken breast
8 oz steak	3 cloves garlic
4 oz shrimp	1 Onion
1 bag of mixed frozen vegetables (california blend)	

1. Prep your vegetables and meats: Slice the onions into slivers or dice them depending on your preference. Slice your steak and chicken into bite size pieces.
2. Marinate your meats (not shrimp) in the soy sauce for at least 2 hours and up to 24 hours.
3. Bring vegetable oil up to medium high heat in frying pan.

4. Press the garlic and combine it with onions and add to oil. Cook until translucent.
5. Add frozen vegetables and meat with marinade.
6. Cook for about 5 minutes until vegetables are the desired consistency.
7. Add hot sauce and cook for 1 more minute, stirring often.
8. Serves 4 (4 oz of meat per person, adjust meat depending on number of servings)

Final thoughts: You can serve this meal as a mixed grill or choose whatever meats you want. I find the variety of meats to be great when you are only getting 4 ounces. You an add scallops, pork, salmon, or swordfish.

Make sure you use your favorite brand of hot sauce, as this is a very personal choice. I love Frank's Red Hot, but you need to use your hot sauce. If you aren't sure what your favorite brand is, ask wherever you normally get your wings and use that.

As well, use as many vegetables as you can. You might have to start slow, with less vegetables until you get used to them. You can use the frozen bagged vegetables or fresh vegetables, or you can use a combination of both.

If you really want to make this like hot wings, you can always add a little dash of dipping sauce, such as the raita, tzaziki or healthy ranch on page 210.

NOTHING SAYS SUMMER TO ME MORE THAN BARBECUING SKEWERS OF MEAT. AS WELL, COOKING MEAT WITH VEGETABLES GETS KIDS USED TO THE FLAVOR OF VEGETABLES. MAKE THE SHISH KABOB PART OF YOUR WEEKLY FOOD CHOICES. THESE CAN BE COOKED IN THE OVEN AS WELL AS ON A BARBECUE.

Shish Kabob

1/2 cup olive oil	1/4 cup soy sauce
1/4 cup white wine vinegar	8 tsp. lemon juice
1 tsp. basil	1/2 tsp. oregano
1 tsp. thyme	1/2 tsp. sage
3 cloves garlic	4 oz. of meat per serving.
3 tomatoes	1 green pepper
1 yellow pepper	1 red onion
1 sweet onion	

1. Mix the spices, olive oil, soy sauce, lemon juice and vinegar.
2. Cut the meat and vegetables into skewer size cubes and pieces.
3. You can marinate the meat in pieces and then put on skewers, or skewer up the meats and

vegetables and then marinate. It depends on how big a container you have to marinate the food and how much space you have in your fridge. Marinate for 2 to 24 hours.

4. Grill the meat over medium heat on a barbecue or in an oven.

5. Serve.

Final thoughts: I vary the meats and vegetables on my skewers. You would be amazed how far the meat will go when you do this. Enough meat for 2 skewers can make 8 skewers when you alternate the meats and vegetables.

I have a bunch of steel skewers in my kitchen, but if you don't, bamboo skewers work well, just remember to soak them in water for up to a day before cooking.

THIS COULD BE ONE OF MY FAVORITE MEALS ON EARTH. FLANK STEAK, PROPERLY MARINATED AND COOKED OVER AN OPEN FIRE IS INCREDIBLE. MY FRIEND ERIC HAS A MARINADE FOR FLANK STEAK THAT IS TO DIE FOR AS WELL. HE HAS BEEN COOKING THIS MEAL SINCE HE WAS IN ELEMENTARY SCHOOL AND WOULD BRING A CONTAINER OF MARINATED STEAK ON CAMPING TRIPS.

Marinated Flank Steak Wraps (with Grilled Vegetables)

1/4 cup olive oil	4 cloves of garlic
1/8 cup soy sauce	1 tbsp chili powder
16 oz flank steak	1/8 cup lemon juice
4 large whole wheat tortillas	salsa
guacamole	

1. Crush your garlic and add it to olive oil, soy sauce and lemon juice.
2. Add the chili powder.
3. Marinate over night.
4. Cook to desired doneness on the barbecue.
5. Warm your tortillas in the microwave with a damp paper towel or over an element on your stove.
6. Stuff each tortilla with 4 ounces of meat, tons of grilled vegetables, salsa and guacamole.

7. Serves 4 (4 oz of meat per person, 1 tortilla)

Final thoughts: Tortillas are really dense bread products, so I don't recommend eating more than 1 large or 2 small tortillas with any meal. Get a fork when you serve yourself and you can put some of the fillings on the side and eat them straight without the wrap.

You can eat some corn in the tortilla or on the side as well. This meal tastes incredible so add as many vegetables as you can and you will still end up full and incredibly satisfied.

Feel free to add more chili powder and even some hot red pepper flakes to spice this meal up if you like.

If you like your flank steak mild or as a non-wrap option, you can leave out the chili powder and instead add 1 tablespoon of capers to the marinade.

THESE VEGETABLES TASTE SO GOOD. IF YOU AREN'T A FAN OF VEGETABLES, THERE IS A GOOD CHANCE THAT THESE WILL WIN YOU OVER TO EATING THEM. WHEN YOU COOK THEM, MAKE TONS BECAUSE THEY GO WELL WITH EVERYTHING.

Grilled Vegetables

1 red onion	1 sweet onion
2 tomatoes	1 yellow pepper
1 orange pepper	1 green pepper
1 teaspoon italian spices	1/8 cup red wine vinegar
1/8 cup olive oil	

1. Slice up the peppers, tomatoes and onions into bite size pieces.
2. Put in a bowl with olive oil, red wine and spices and toss .
3. Marinate up to one hour.
4. Barbecue until the peppers are slightly blackened, about 10 minutes on medium heat.
5. Serve.

Final thoughts: There are many ways to prepare these vegetables, including large slices grilled directly on the barbecue, smaller slices on a skewer, or my favorite, even smaller bites in a barbecue basket, just remember to stir, flip or turn your vegetables regularly.

I cannot stress enough how good these vegetables taste the day after as well. I eat them in my denver omelette (see recipe above) as well as a topping for 4 ounces of steak. These would be great on home made pizza as well.

SALMON IS GREAT FOR YOU AND TASTES GREAT.
EATING SALMON WITH STEAMED VEGETABLES AND
MAYBE SOME CANNED CORN OR PEAS IS A VERY
HEALTHY, VERY SATISFYING MEAL.

Salmon (with steamed vegetables)

4 - 4 oz salmon filets or	2 cups soy sauce
1 - 16 oz side of salmon	1 tsp. lime juice
1 clove garlic	pepper
2 tsp sesame oil	1 tbsp rice vinegar

1. Mix the ingredients and marinate for 15 minutes.
2. Place skin side down to a grill on medium heat.
3. Brush with remaining marinade.
4. Grill for about 20 minutes, until fish flakes easily.
5. Serves 4.

Final thoughts: The cooking of fish can be a little tricky. I think excellent salmon is cooked to a medium rare, but many people overcook their salmon. Getting very good at cooking salmon can be the sign of an excellent chef.

This can be cooked in the oven as well, so you can make it easily, year round. Line a baking pan with tin foil. Roast in a 450 degree oven for about 10 minutes, brushing with the marinade about 5 minutes in.

I love the flavor of sesame oil, but it is quite a powerful taste that it might take you awhile to get used to it. You can use olive oil if you prefer or if you don't have any sesame oil.

If you don't have any rice vinegar use twice the lime juice. If you don't have lime, use lemon.

You can add some shredded green onions on top when you serve this dish to make it look quite gourmet. You can also add some sesame seeds.

Finally, you can turn this marinade into a glaze if you want. It takes a bit of sugar to do this, but it makes a great meal. You can do this by adding about 1/4 cup of maple syrup. Maple syrup is probably the best sweetener you can use. If you don't have any maple syrup use 2 tablespoons of brown sugar. When glazing, set aside a small amount of the marinade before you marinade the fish. Add the sugar or maple syrup to this. Remove the salmon from wherever you were cooking it, brush it with the glaze and move the salmon into an oven on a high broil (500° F) for 2 to 3 minutes. If you are adding sesame seeds, add them before moving the salmon to the broiler.

THIS ISN'T THE BEST VEGETABLE DISH IN THE WORLD, BUT IT COULD BE THE EASIEST. I ADD THIS TO MANY MEATS AND IT DOES THE TRICK.

Steamed Vegetables

1 bag frozen mixed vegetables	2 tbsp soy sauce
2 tbsp water	

1. Pour as much frozen vegetables that you plan to eat into a bowl.
2. Add soy sauce and water .
3. Put in microwave on high for 2 minutes or until done to your desired level.
4. Serve.

Final thoughts: There are many different blends of vegetables. I like the what is typically referred to as a california blend and the asian blend. It is great to have a couple of bags of these in the freezer. Remember though, these aren't the best vegetables and fresh is generally better, so if you can, prepare your own blends.

SAUCES

Sauces are so good and can make a meal, the problem is that they can ruin any attempt to eat healthy. If you can develop a few healthier sauces and use these sparingly, you may not even notice that you are eating healthier.

I ONLY RECENTLY DISCOVERED RAITA. IT IS AN INDIAN VERSION OF TZAZIKI AND IT IS JUST AS TASTY. WHEN YOU ARE EATING INDIAN FOODS, THIS COOLING YOGURT BASED DIP OR TOPPING IS SO VERY WELCOME!

Raita

2 cups plain greek yogurt	1/2 tsp. salt
1/2 tsp. black pepper 1	1 cup grated carrots (parboiled)
/2 tsp. ground roast cumin seeds	

1. Mix all of the ingredients and transfer to a serving bowl.

Final thoughts: There are many different Raita recipes so experiment. When you find one you like at a local indian restaurant, be sure to ask them how they make it. I have found that people are very willing to share their recipes when you genuinely appreciate what they have made.

I AM A TZAZIKI ADDICT. I ABSOLUTELY LOVE THIS STUFF. IF I AM EATING A SOUVLAKI MEAL I DROWN THE SKEWERS IN TZAZIKI. THIS IS ONE OF THE GREAT DIPS OF ALL TIME.

Tzaziki

2 cups plain greek yogurt	4 cloves of garlic
1 cucumber	2 pinches salt

1. Peel the cucumber, seed and grate it using a standard cheese grater. Drain the cucumber in a cheesecloth or coffee filter. Sprinkle a pinch or two of salt on the cucumber and Let it dry.
2. Mix the ingredients.
3. Refrigerate the tzaziki for at least one hour before serving.

Final thoughts: I never drain the cucumber and end up with a pretty watery sauce. It is a good idea to take the time to strain it. If you don't use greek yogurt, you will need to strain the yogurt as well. Use a coffee filter and let it drain for one hour. Taking the time with tzaziki is really worth it. This may not be the easiest sauce, but it could be the tastiest.

RANCH IS HARD TO BEAT. IT IS A GREAT DIPPING SAUCE, BUT IT IS USUALLY A PRETTY HIGH FAT SAUCE OR DRESSING. I MAKE MINE USING GREEK YOGURT.

Healthy Ranch

2 cups plain greek yogurt	2 tsp ranch dressing mix
1/4 tsp Cayenne pepper (opt)	

1. Mix.
2. Serve.

Final thoughts: This is a great sauce without the cayenne pepper, but it totally comes to life when you add the pepper. Try it, you will love it. With the pepper I call it spicy yogurt dip.

Personal Measurements:

First Measurements:

Blood Pressure		MM/DD/YYYY
Cholesterol:	Total	MM/DD/YYYY
	LDL	
	HDL	
	Serum	
Waist To Hip:		MM/DD/YYYY
Weight:		MM/DD/YYYY
Fat %		MM/DD/YYYY
Resting HR		MM/DD/YYYY

End of Chapter 7 Measurements:

Blood Pressure		MM/DD/YYYY
Cholesterol:	Total	MM/DD/YYYY
	LDL	
	HDL	
	Serum	
Waist To Hip:		MM/DD/YYYY
Weight:		MM/DD/YYYY
Fat %		MM/DD/YYYY
Resting HR		MM/DD/YYYY

Notes: